The Handbook of
Diabetes Mellitus and Cardiovascular Disease

Steven P Marso, Editor

The Mid America Heart Institute
Kansas City, Missouri, USA

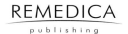

REMEDICA
publishing

LONDON • CHICAGO

Contributors

Robert AS Ariëns, PhD
Academic Unit of Molecular Vascular Medicine
University of Leeds School of Medicine
G-Floor, Martin Wing
The General Infirmary
Leeds LS1 3EX, UK

Deepak L Bhatt, MD
Staff, Interventional Cardiology
Program Director, Interventional Cardiology Fellowship
The Cleveland Clinic Foundation
Department of Cardiovascular Medicine/Desk F25
9500 Euclid Avenue
Cleveland, Ohio 44195, USA

Peter J Grant, MD, FRCP
Academic Unit of Molecular Vascular Medicine
University of Leeds School of Medicine
G-Floor, Martin Wing
The General Infirmary
Leeds LS1 3EX, UK

Steven P Marso, MD, FACC
The Mid America Heart Institute
Saint Luke's Hospital
4401 Wornall, Kansas City
Missouri 64111, USA

Th
D
al
D

Remedica State of the Art series
ISSN 1472-4626

Also available
Management of Atherosclerotic Carotid Disease
Management of Peripheral Arterial Disease
Rheumatoid Arthritis
Viral Co-infections in HIV
Kidney Transplantation

Forthcoming titles
Inflammatory Bowel Disease
Multiple Myeloma

Published by the Remedica Group
32–38 Osnaburgh Street, London, NW1 3ND, UK
Remedica Inc, Tri-State International Center, Building 25, Suite 150, Lincolnshire, IL 60069, USA

Tel: +44 20 7388 7677
Fax: +44 20 7388 7457
Email: books@remedica.com
www.remedica.com

Publisher: Andrew Ward
In-house editors: Roisin O'Brien and Catherine Harris

© 2003 Remedica Publishing Limited

ISBN 1 901346 59 5
British Library Cataloguing-in Publication Data
A catalogue record for this book is available from the British Library

Darren K McGuire, MD, MHSc
The Donald W Reynolds Cardiovascular Research Center
University of Texas Southwestern Medical Center at Dallas
5323 Harry Hines Boulevard
Dallas, Texas 75390–9047, USA

Joel P Reginelli, MD
The Cleveland Clinic Foundation
Department of Cardiovascular Medicine/Desk F25
9500 Euclid Avenue
Cleveland, Ohio 44195, USA

Matthew T Roe, MD, MHS
Division of Cardiology
Duke Clinical Research Institute
Duke University Medical Center
Durham, North Carolina 27710, USA

David M Safley, MD
University of Missouri – Kansas City
Mid America Heart Institute
Saint Luke's Hospital
4401 Wornall, Kansas City
Missouri 64111, USA

Benjamin H Trichon, MD
Division of Cardiology
Duke Clinical Research Institute
Duke University Medical Center
Durham, North Carolina 27710, USA

Acknowledgements

I would like to thank Deborah J Spiers for her expert assistance.

Preface

The management of diabetes mellitus is a global concern. Few disease states are as common or have the health implications of diabetes. Although diabetes is a disorder of the "insulin–glucose axis", the major pathobiology occurs in the vascular system. It is quite clear in the modern era of medicine that the primary cause of mortality and major morbidity is directly attributable to both macrovascular and microvascular complications. In fact, 70% of all case fatalities are a net result of a cardiovascular complication. Additionally, the percentage of the world population affected with type 2 diabetes is increasing at an alarming rate. Although initially thought to be a disease of developed nations, the vast majority of new cases over the next 20 years are predicted to emerge in developing countries. Given the financial burden and the requisite clinical infrastructure needed to treat this high-risk population, major efforts will be required to provide adequate care. Furthermore, with the globalization of diabetes, it is fundamental that healthcare providers are kept up-to-date with the latest in disease management strategies. This handbook provides a concise, to-the-point, pragmatic approach, which will make the provision of optimal care in patients with diabetes possible.

Steven P Marso
Mid America Heart Institute

Contents

1

Epidemiology of diabetes mellitus and cardiovascular disease

Darren K McGuire & Sunil V Rao

Introduction

As a result of an aging, increasingly obese, and decreasingly physically active population, the global incidence and prevalence of diabetes mellitus is exploding [1–3]. This is due almost exclusively to an increase in type 2 diabetes mellitus (T2DM); T2DM represents more than 90% of all cases of the disease. The medical and public health challenges are further compounded by the observation that diabetic patients have a considerable risk for cardiovascular disease (CVD); up to 80% of deaths within this high-risk population are due to CVD [4].

This chapter reviews the epidemiology of T2DM and the associated cardiovascular complications. Although the incidence of diabetes will continue to increase within the industrialized nations, the predominant increase in the number of new cases will be in developing countries.

Epidemiology of diabetes mellitus

The World Health Organization (WHO) has projected that the prevalence of diabetes will double over the next 22 years – from a current figure of 150 million to an estimated 300 million people by the year 2025 [2]. It is likely that these figures are a gross underestimation of the problem, given that as many as half of affected patients remain undiagnosed [4–6].

United States

NHANES (the National Health and Nutrition Examination Survey) II and III examined the prevalence of diabetes among a population-based sample of American adults [4,7]. Over the 18 years spanning these two epidemiologic studies (1976–1994), the estimated prevalence of diabetes among the US adult population has increased from 6.6% to 7.8%. Although the absolute increase on a percentage basis is relatively small, when the rapidly expanding US population is taken into account, this represents almost a doubling of the number of patients with diabetes – from 8 million to an estimated 15.6 million people [4,7].

By extrapolating the NHANES data, the US Centers for Disease Control and Prevention estimated that 8.6% of US adults currently have diabetes, and projected an annual incidence of new diagnoses of T2DM of 625,000 [8].

As the seventh leading reported cause of death in the US, diabetes consumes an inordinate proportion of healthcare resources and is associated with a doubling of annual per capita expenditure [9]. Diabetic patients have an increased likelihood of premature discontinuation of gainful employment and a 3-fold higher rate of disability claims than people without diabetes [10].

Worldwide

Over the next few decades, the greatest anticipated increase in diabetes will come from developing countries (see **Figure 1**) [2]. By the year 2025, it is expected that the worldwide prevalence of diabetes will affect 5.4% of the adult population, with 75% of these cases in developing countries [2]. This will primarily be a result of decreasing rates of physical activity, an increasing prevalence of obesity, and an increasing consumption of high-caloric diets [11].

For example, the prevalence of diabetes tripled in China between 1986 and 1996 [12], and an additional doubling of the Chinese diabetic population is expected over the next 2 decades – from 16 million currently to an estimated 38 million people by 2020 [2].

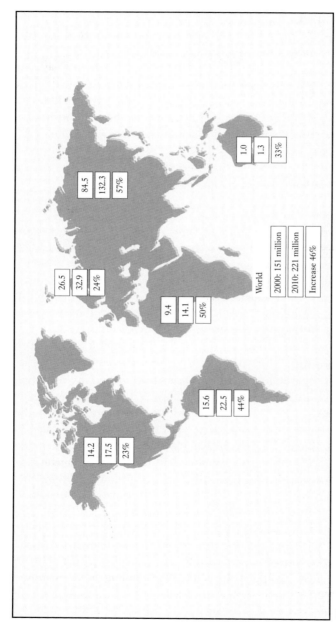

Figure 1. Numbers of people with diabetes (in millions) in 2000 and 2010 estimate (top and middle values, respectively), and the percentage increase. Reprinted with permission from: Zimmet P, Alberti KG, Shaw J. Global and societal implications of the diabetes epidemic. *Nature* 2001;414:782–7.

Likewise, India has the largest and fastest growing diabetic population in the world; the current figure of 19.4 million is expected to increase to over 57 million people by 2025 [2].

The increase in life expectancy in developing countries – as well as an evolving lifestyle predisposed to obesity and diabetes – contributes to the increasing prevalence of the disease; the risk for diabetes is greater with advancing age and patients with diabetes are living longer.

Special populations at risk for diabetes

The elderly
The world's population is aging, and the elderly are disproportionately affected by diabetes [2–4,13]. For example, data from NHANES III demonstrated that the prevalence of diabetes ranged from 1.6% in men aged 20–39 years to 21.1% in men older than 75 years [7]. It is expected that the aging global population will account for at least half of the projected increase in the prevalence of diabetes in coming years [8].

Ethnic groups
Diabetes is a particular risk among certain ethnic groups, including African Americans, Asians, Hispanics, and Native Americans (see **Figure 2**) [4,14–16]. Over the next 50 years, 35% of the projected increase in newly diagnosed cases of diabetes in the US will be attributable to the increasing proportion of minorities in the population [17]. This association is most likely a result of complex interactions between genetic predisposition and environmental influences.

Children
There are few epidemiologic data on the incidence and prevalence of T2DM specifically in children, but due to the decrease in physical activity and the increase in obesity among children around the world, there has been a steady increase in the prevalence of T2DM among this historically low-risk population [18].

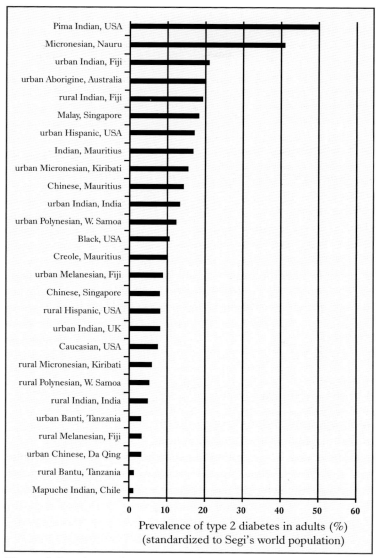

Figure 2. Prevalence of type 2 diabetes in selected populations. Adapted with permission from: Zimmet PZ, McCarty DJ, de Courten MP. The global epidemiology of noninsulin-dependent diabetes mellitus and the metabolic syndrome. *J Diabetes Complications* 1997;11:60–8.

1997 ADA	1999 WHO
Symptoms (polyuria, polydipsia, or weight loss) AND a random glucose ≥200 mg/dL (11.1 mmol/L)	FPG ≥126 mg/dL (7.0 mmol/L)
	OR
OR	2-hour postload plasma glucose ≥200 mg/dL (11.1 mmol/L)
FPG ≥126 mg/dL (7.0 mmol/L)	
OR	
75-g OGTT 2-hour glucose >200 mg/dL (not recommended for routine clinical use)	

Table 1. Diagnostic criteria for diabetes according to the American Diabetes Association (ADA) and the World Health Organization (WHO) [20,123]. FPG: fasting plasma glucose; OGTT: oral glucose tolerance testing.

The global variation in the prevalence of type 1 diabetes (T1DM) varies from 0.7 per 100,000 people in Shanghai to over 35 per 100,000 people in Finland; 120,000 individuals under the age of 18 years have T1DM [19]. Although T1DM accounts for a small minority of diabetes cases overall, these cases represent the majority of patients affected by diabetes under the age of 19 years.

Factors contributing to the pandemic of diabetes

Modification of diagnostic criteria

Both the American Diabetes Association (ADA) and the WHO have liberalized the diagnostic criteria for glucose intolerance and diabetes over the last decade [20]. The WHO criteria are based on both the fasting plasma glucose (FPG) level and the result from oral glucose tolerance testing (OGTT), whereas the ADA criteria rely primarily on the FPG level (see **Table 1**) [21]. While the WHO criteria are more sensitive [22], the ADA criteria are more broadly applicable given the ubiquitous testing of FPG and the uncommon practice of subjecting patients to a 2-hour glucose tolerance test.

Aging population

Increased life expectancy has led to an increase in the number of people over 65 years of age in both the developed and developing worlds [23]. By the year 2020, 12.9% of the world's population is expected be over the age of 60 years, compared with 9.9% in the year 2000 [24]. Due to the clear association between age and the development of diabetes, this increase in the number of older individuals in the population will inevitably contribute to the increased prevalence of diabetes.

Obesity

In both developed and developing countries, obesity – which is directly associated with the development of insulin resistance, glucose intolerance, and diabetes (see **Table 2**) [25,26] – is increasing at an alarming rate [27–29]. For example, in the US, results from NHANES III (1988–1991) demonstrated that approximately two thirds of the adult population was overweight and, of these, approximately 33% were obese. This is a 25% increase compared with data from 10 years earlier [28]. Also in the NHANES III cohort, 67% of those with T2DM were overweight, and almost half were obese [30]. While the mechanism by which obesity contributes to glucose intolerance remains elusive, it is likely to be a combination of genetic factors and molecular mechanisms in which skeletal myocytes and adipocytes play a role [31–33].

Decreasing levels of physical activity

Leisure-time physical activity is continuing to decrease worldwide, resulting in an increasingly sedentary population and greater risk for diabetes [11]. Data from the Nurses' Health Study suggested that modest physical activity is associated with a decreased risk for developing diabetes [34]. Subsequent randomized trials have proven the effectiveness of lifestyle modification for diabetes prevention [35,36]. In addition to weight management, physical activity is directly associated with improved glycometabolism – as demonstrated by decreased insulin levels, increased insulin sensitivity, and a lower incidence of diabetes [37–39].

Body-mass index	Cases	Person-years of follow-up	Age-standardized incidence rate*	Age-adjusted relative risk (95% CI)
kg/m²	n		%	
<22.0	55	466,052	13.0	1.0 (reference)
22.0–22.9	71	194,433	37.4	2.9 (2.0–4.1)
23.0–23.9	88	156,770	54.9	4.3 (3.1–5.8)
24.0–24.9	94	142,392	62.9	5.0 (3.6–6.6)
25.0–26.9	227	198,484	103.5	8.1 (6.2–10.5)
27.0–28.9	267	119,662	200.4	15.8 (12.7–19.8)
29.0–30.9	329	84,880	354.5	27.6 (22.7–33.5)
31.0–32.9	263	47,119	521.2	40.3 (33.7–48.3)
33.0–34.9	224	29,885	703.6	54.0 (45.6–64.0)
≥35.0	579	46,636	1190.5	93.2 (81.4–106.6)

*Rate per 100,000 persons standardized to the age distribution of length of follow-up in the cohort.

Table 2. Association between body-mass index and prevalence of type 2 diabetes. Adapted with permission from: Colditz GA, Willett WC, Rotnitzky A et al. Weight gain as a risk factor for clinical diabetes mellitus in women. *Ann Intern Med* 1995;122:481–6.

Diet

Other lifestyle factors – such as diets low in dietary fiber with a high glycemic load [40], and high-fat diets – have also been associated with the development of diabetes [41]. An analysis of 42,504 subjects in the Physicians' Health Study found a relative risk of 1.59 for developing diabetes with the consumption of a diet high in fat [42]. Similarly, in the Nurses' Health Study, an increased intake of dietary cereal fiber, whole grain foods, and trans-fatty acids, with a decreased intake of saturated fat, was associated with a 33%–50% reduced risk of developing T2DM [43,44].

Prevention of diabetes mellitus

Targeted interventions are being developed to prevent T2DM among high-risk groups, including obese and sedentary individuals, people with a family history of T2DM, and those with documented abnormalities in glucose metabolism not meeting the diagnostic criteria for diabetes.

Lifestyle modification – including diet, weight loss, and physical activity prescription – has been shown to be effective for preventing (or at least delaying) the onset of diabetes; up to a 60% relative reduction in risk is associated with such interventions [35,36,45,46].

Pharmacologic therapies – including metformin [46], acarbose [47], ramipril and captopril [48,49], troglitazone [50], and losartan [51] – also decrease the risk of incident diabetes among high-risk cohorts. However, most of these agents are associated with a more modest 25%–30% reduction in risk of incident diabetes, much lower than the reduction observed with therapeutic lifestyle modifications. Studies are presently underway to directly test the effect of many of these drugs on the risk for diabetes in prospective clinical investigations.

Epidemiology of diabetic cardiovascular disease

Macrovascular disease (myocardial infarction [MI], stroke, and peripheral arterial disease [PAD]) accounts for the majority of morbidity and mortality associated with T2DM (see **Figure 3**) [52–56]. For example, UKPDS (the United Kingdom Prospective Diabetes Study) showed that the 10-year risk for all macrovascular complications was more than 4-times higher than the corresponding risk for microvascular complications within diabetic patients [57].

Diabetes confers a long-term cardiovascular risk similar to that observed among patients without diabetes but who have had a prior MI (see **Table 3**) [58]. Once coronary artery disease (CAD) develops, diabetes doubles the risk for acute coronary syndromes, with an additional doubling of clinical risk once these events occur [59–61]. Despite these reported observations, a survey of 2,008 diabetic subjects conducted by the ADA and the American College of Cardiology revealed that nearly 70% did not believe that CVD was a serious risk associated with diabetes.

Ischemic heart disease

The most common cause of death among patients with diabetes is ischemic heart disease [62,63]. Patients with diabetes also have poorer clinical outcomes than nondiabetic patients after acute coronary syndromes, including ST-segment elevation MI [64–66] and non-ST-segment elevation acute coronary syndromes (see **Figure 4**) [60,61]. Likewise, after adjusting for other factors, the Framingham study documented significantly higher mortality and a higher rate of reinfarction and heart failure for patients with diabetes in the acute and postinfarction period [67].

Congestive heart failure

The most common cause of congestive heart failure (CHF) in the US is ischemic heart disease, and this is especially true for patients with diabetes [68]. However, after adjusting for the prevalence of CAD, diabetes remains an independent predictor for CHF [69] and

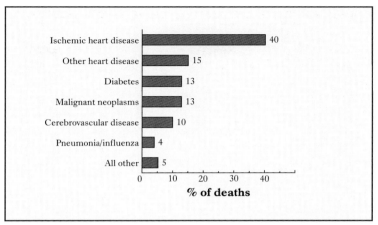

Figure 3. Causes of death among patients with diabetes. Adapted with permission from: Geiss LS, Herman WH, Smith PJ. Mortality in non-insulin dependent diabetes. In: Harris M, ed. *Diabetes in America.* 2nd ed. Bethesda, MD: National Institute of Diabetes and Digestive and Kidney Diseases, 1995:233–55.

an independent predictor of mortality among patients with CHF [70]. The independent association between diabetes and risk for CHF associated with diabetes has been demonstrated across the entire spectrum of acute coronary syndromes [60,66,71,72].

Cerebrovascular disease
Hypertension and dyslipidemia commonly coexist with diabetes, conferring a high risk of stroke. However, even after adjusting for these factors, diabetes remains an independent predictor for ischemic neurologic events, suggesting the contribution of additional diabetes-related factors [53,73].

Peripheral vascular disease
Peripheral vascular disease (PVD) affects up to 17% of patients with diabetes [74] and is associated with lower-extremity ulceration, gangrene, and amputation. The distribution of PVD in patients with diabetes differs from that in the nondiabetic population: the distal lower-extremity arterial circulation is more

11

Event	Nondiabetic subjects			Subjects with type 2 diabetes			All subjects	
	Prior MI (n=69)	No prior MI (n=1304)	P value	Prior MI (n=169)	No prior MI (n=890)	P value	P value for prior MI vs. no prior MI	P value for diabetes vs. no diabetes
Fatal or nonfatal MI								
Incidence during follow-up	18.8	3.5	<0.001	45.0	20.2	<0.001	<0.001	<0.001
Events/100 person-years	3.0	0.5		7.8	3.2			
Fatal or nonfatal stroke								
Incidence during follow-up	7.2	1.9	0.01	19.5	10.3	<0.001	<0.001	<0.001
Events/100 person-years	1.2	0.3		3.4	1.6			
Death from cardiovascular causes								
Incidence during follow-up	15.9	2.1	<0.001	42.0	15.4	<0.001	<0.001	<0.001
Events/100 person-years	2.6	0.3		7.3	2.5			

*P values were calculated with Cox proportional-hazards models. The Cox models were adjusted for age and sex. MI denotes myocardial infarction.

Table 3. Probability of myocardial infarction over a 7-year period according to diabetes status among patients with and without prior myocardial infarction (MI). Adapted with permission from: Haffner SM, Lehto S, Ronnemaa T et al. Mortality from coronary heart disease in subjects with type 2 diabetes and in nondiabetic subjects with and without prior myocardial infarction. *N Engl J Med* 1998;339:229–34.

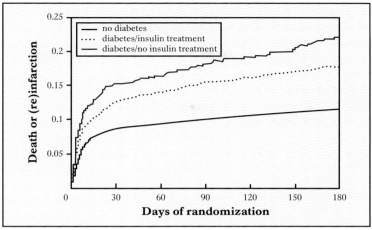

Figure 4. The probability of death or myocardial infarction within the 6 months following an acute coronary syndrome episode according to diabetes status, with and without insulin requirement. Reprinted with permission from: McGuire DK, Emanuelsson H, Granger CB et al. Influence of diabetes mellitus on clinical outcomes across the spectrum of acute coronary syndromes. Findings from the GUSTO-IIb study. GUSTO IIb Investigators. *Eur Heart J* 2000;21:1750–8.

affected in patients with diabetes, while nondiabetic patients tend to have more proximal disease [75]. The distal disease of diabetes often precludes effective revascularization, resulting in higher rates of amputation.

In addition to limb loss, diabetic patients with PVD experience a 70%–80% higher mortality compared with diabetic patients who do not have PVD [76,77]. Risk factors associated with the development of PVD and lower-extremity ulceration include: male gender; a longer than 10-year duration of diabetes; poor glucose control; a requirement for insulin; and the presence of cardiovascular, retinal, or renal complications [78].

Hypertension
Hypertension affects up to 70% of patients with diabetes, contributing significantly to the associated cardiovascular and

renal complications [54,79]. Increasing age, male sex, a longer duration of diabetes, poor glycemic control (defined as the percentage of glycosylated hemoglobin), and proteinuria are independent predictors of hypertension [80].

Dyslipidemia

Lipid abnormalities in T2DM develop concomitantly with the failure of insulin activity leading to the release of fatty acids from adipose tissue, increased delivery of free-fatty acids to the liver, and increased hepatic synthesis of very low-density lipoproteins (VLDL) [81–83]. This abnormal lipid profile – characterized by normal or modestly elevated low-density lipoprotein (LDL) cholesterol, low high-density lipoprotein (HDL) cholesterol, high triglycerides (TGs), and a preponderance of small, dense LDL particles – is associated with a markedly increased cardiovascular risk among diabetic patients [83–85].

The degree of TG elevation is directly related to the degree of glucose intolerance and glucose control [86], with lesser effect of glucose parameters on HDL and LDL concentrations. Pooling of unpublished data from the ADA, NHANES II, the Rancho Bernardo California Diabetes Study, the Japanese-American Study of Diabetes, the San Antonio Texas Heart Study, and the San Luis Valley Study shows that among patients with diabetes, mean total cholesterol and HDL levels are higher in women (total cholesterol: 238 mg/dL, HDL: 49–55 mg/dL) than in men (total cholesterol: 223 mg/dL, HDL: 42–45 mg/dL) [86].

Prevention of cardiovascular complications in diabetes

Despite the prevalence of diabetes and the associated cardiovascular risk, few studies have specifically examined the effect of medical therapies and interventions among this high-risk population of patients. Most of the available data in this area derive from epidemiologic observations and subgroup analyses of clinical trial data.

Epidemiologic data have clearly demonstrated a correlation between the glycometabolic state and clinical risk [87–90], though the effect of glycemic control on cardiovascular risk has yet to be definitively established [57,91–93]. UKPDS demonstrated a beneficial effect of intensive glycemic control versus "usual care" on a composite endpoint of diabetic complications [57], but this effect was much more modest than expected (35.3% vs. 38.5%, relative risk [RR] reduction: 12%), and the trial was underpowered to evaluate the effects of such a strategy specifically on cardiovascular risk. Furthermore, it appears that the strategy used for glycemic control may be more important than the degree of control achieved.

A prospective, randomized substudy of the UKPDS demonstrated the superiority of metformin compared with either insulin or sulfonylureas for cardiovascular risk modification [94]. Likewise, the DIGAMI (Diabetes Mellitus, Insulin Glucose Infusion in Acute Myocardial Infarction) study demonstrated a 1-year mortality benefit of acute intravenous hyperinsulinemic/hyperglycemic treatment followed by chronic subcutaneous insulin therapy, as opposed to usual care among patients presenting with an acute coronary syndrome (18.6% vs. 26.1%, RR reduction: 29%)[95].

Although the role of glycemic control and the merits of various hypoglycemic strategies remain to be defined with regard to cardiovascular risk modification, several treatments have been associated with marked improvement in the clinical outcome among subsets of patients with diabetes enrolled in cardiovascular randomized clinical trials in both the primary and secondary prevention settings.

A number of therapies for primary and secondary cardiovascular risk modification have been demonstrated to be particularly effective among diabetic patients. These include antiplatelet therapy (aspirin and/or clopidogrel) [96–100], angiotensin-converting enzyme (ACE) inhibitors [101–104], beta-blockers [104], thiazide diuretics [49,105], and the 3-hydroxy-3-

methylglutaryl-coenzyme A (HMG-CoA) reductase inhibitors (statins) [106–109].

Based on these data, clinical practice guidelines recommend:

- consideration of aspirin (or clopidogrel) and ACE inhibitor use for all patients with diabetes [110,111]

- statin therapy (with therapeutic lipid targets identical to the targets in the population with CAD) for patients with dyslipidemia [112]

- administration of beta-blockers, ACE inhibitors, and thiazide diuretics – with aggressive blood pressure targets – for patients with hypertension [113]

More recently, losartan – an angiotensin receptor blocker (ARB) – was shown to be superior to atenolol for cardiovascular risk reduction (composite endpoint of cardiovascular death, MI, and stroke) among patients with hypertension and left ventricular hypertrophy in a large-scale randomized trial. An exaggerated treatment benefit was observed among the diabetic cohort treated with losartan versus placebo (17.6% vs. 22.8%, RR reduction: 24%) [114]. The effect of combining ARB treatment with ACE inhibitors or beta-blockers remains unknown.

Similarly, the potent antiplatelet effect of the glycoprotein (GP)IIb/IIIa antagonists is particularly effective in the setting of diabetes for patients with acute coronary syndromes [115–118] and those undergoing percutaneous coronary intervention [119].

Cardiovascular complications account for the majority of the increased morbidity and mortality associated with T2DM. Therefore, a primary therapeutic goal should be to improve cardiovascular clinical outcomes in these high-risk patients. Until more definitive data regarding the impact of current hypoglycemic strategies on important clinical outcomes are available, it is critical that some of the focus of therapy should be directed away from the achievement of glycemic control and towards the aggressive modification of cardiovascular risk.

Conclusion

Diabetes is a prevalent disease with the number of cases increasing at an alarming rate. Review of current literature suggests that the elderly and individuals from ethnic minorities will be disproportionately affected in the future, and the increasing rate of diabetes among children demands particular attention. Worldwide, the aging of the population and industrialization of developing countries will contribute to the increased prevalence of this disease.

The major cause of morbidity and mortality associated with diabetes is from atherosclerotic macrovascular disease – such as peripheral, cerebrovascular, and CAD. As the prevalence of diabetes continues to rise, the concomitant increases in these diseases will inevitably strain healthcare resources.

So far, the only interventions that have proven effective at reducing the macrovascular disease complications associated with diabetes are those that modify coexisting risk factors such as aberrant lifestyles, obesity, dyslipidemia, and hypertension. Disappointingly, strategies to target glycemic metabolism improvements have had little effect on the cardiovascular risk.

The myriad of cardiovascular complications associated with diabetes will make this disease a public health emergency in the foreseeable future. Therefore, the development of new strategies aimed at both primary prevention of diabetes and the prevention of diabetic complications will remain important research and clinical objectives.

References

1. Eschwege E, Simon D, Balkau B. The growing burden of diabetes in the world population. *International Diabetes Federation Bulletin* 1997;42:14–9.
2. King H, Aubert RE, Herman WH. Global burden of diabetes, 1995–2025: prevalence, numerical estimates, and projections. *Diabetes Care* 1998;21:1414–31.
3. Boyle JP, Honeycutt AA, Narayan KM et al. Projection of diabetes burden through 2050: impact of changing demography and disease prevalence in the US. *Diabetes Care* 2001;24:1936–40.
4. Harris MI, Hadden WC, Knowler WC et al. Prevalence of diabetes and impaired glucose tolerance and plasma glucose levels in US population aged 20–74 years. *Diabetes* 1987;36:523–34.
5. Saydah SH, Loria CM, Eberhardt MS et al. Subclinical states of glucose intolerance and risk of death in the US. *Diabetes Care* 2001;24:447–53.
6. Taubert G, Winkelman BR, Schleiffer T et al. Prevalence, predictors, and consequences of unrecognized diabetes mellitus in 3266 patients scheduled for coronary angiography. *Am Heart J* 2003;145:285–91.
7. Harris MI, Flegal KM, Cowie CC et al. Prevalence of diabetes, impaired fasting glucose, and impaired glucose tolerance in US adults. The Third National Health and Nutrition Examination Survey, 1988–1994. *Diabetes Care* 1998;21:518–24.
8. Kenny SJ, Aubert RE, Geiss LS. Prevalence and incidence of non-insulin-dependent diabetes. In: National Diabetes Group, ed. *Diabetes in America*. Bethesda, MD: National Institute of Diabetes and Digestive and Kidney Diseases, 1995:47–68.
9. Ramsey S, Summers KH, Leong SA et al. Productivity and medical costs of diabetes in a large employer population. *Diabetes Care* 2002;25:23–9.
10. Yassin AS, Beckles GL, Messonnier ML. Disability and its economic impact among adults with diabetes. *J Occup Environ Med* 2002;44:136–42.
11. Popkin BM, Horton S, Kim S et al. Trends in diet, nutritional status, and diet-related non-communicable diseases in China and India: the economic costs of the nutrition transition. *Nutr Rev* 2001;59:379–90.
12. Pan XR, Yang WY, Li GW et al. Prevalence of diabetes and its risk factors in China, 1994. National Diabetes Prevention and Control Cooperative Group. *Diabetes Care* 1997; 20:1664–9.
13. Wilson PW, Kannel WB. Obesity, diabetes, and risk of cardiovascular disease in the elderly. *Am J Geriatr Cardiol* 2002;11:119–23.
14. Bassford TL. Health status of Hispanic elders. *Clin Geriatr Med* 1995;11:25–38.
15. Fujimoto WY, Leonetti DL, Kinyoun JL et al. Prevalence of diabetes mellitus and impaired glucose tolerance among second-generation Japanese-American men. *Diabetes* 1987;36:721–9.
16. Knowler WC, Bennett PH, Hamman RF et al. Diabetes incidence and prevalence in Pima Indians: a 19-fold greater incidence than in Rochester, Minnesota. *Am J Epidemiol* 1978;108:497–505.
17. Day JC. Population projections of the US by age, sex, race and Hispanic origin 1995–2050. Washington DC: US Bureau of the Census. Current Population Reports No. 25–1130, 1996.
18. Greger N, Edwin CM. Obesity: a pediatric epidemic. *Pediatr Ann* 2001;30:694–700.
19. LaPorte RE, Matsushima M, Chang YF. Prevalence and incidence of insulin-dependent diabetes. In: National Diabetes Group, ed. *Diabetes in America*. 2nd ed. Bethesda MD: National Institute of Diabetes and Kidney Diseases, 1995:37–46.

20. World Heath Organization. Definition, Diagnosis and Classification of Diabetes Mellitus and Its Complications: Part 1: Report of a WHO Consultation: Diagnosis and Classification of Diabetes Mellitus. Geneva: World Health Organization, 1999.

21. The Expert Committee on the Diagnosis and Classification of Diabetes Mellitus. Report of the Expert Committee on the Diagnosis and Classification of Diabetes Mellitus. *Diabetes Care* 1997;20:1183–97.

22. Harris MI, Eastman RC, Cowie CC et al. Comparison of diabetes diagnostic categories in the US population according to the 1997 American Diabetes Association and 1980–1985 World Health Organization diagnostic criteria. *Diabetes Care* 1997;20:1859–62.

23. Butler RN. Population aging and health. *BMJ* 1997;315:1082–4.

24. Kunugi T. Women and population aging. *Asia Pac Pop J* 1989;4:75–9.

25. Folsom AR, Kushi LH, Anderson KE et al. Associations of general and abdominal obesity with multiple health outcomes in older women: the Iowa Women's Health Study. *Arch Intern Med* 2000;160:2117–28.

26. Brancati FL, Kao WH, Folsom AR et al. Incident type 2 diabetes mellitus in African American and white adults: the Atherosclerosis Risk in Communities Study. *JAMA* 2000;283:2253–9.

27. Kuczmarski RJ, Flegal KM, Campbell SM et al. Increasing prevalence of overweight among US adults. The National Health and Nutrition Examination Surveys, 1960 to 1991. *JAMA* 1994;272:205–11.

28. Flegal KM, Carroll MD, Kuczmarski RJ et al. Overweight and obesity in the United States: prevalence and trends, 1960–1994. *Int J Obes Relat Metab Disord* 1998;22:39–47.

29. James PT, Leach R, Kalamara E et al. The worldwide obesity epidemic. *Obes Res* 2001; 9 (Suppl. 4):228–33S.

30. National Task Force on the Prevention and Treatment of Obesity. Overweight, obesity, and health risk. *Arch Intern Med* 2000;160:898–904.

31. Kahn BB, Flier JS. Obesity and insulin resistance. *J Clin Invest* 2000;106:473–81.

32. Ryder JW, Gilbert M, Zierath JR. Skeletal muscle and insulin sensitivity: pathophysiological alterations. *Front Biosci* 2001;6:D154–63.

33. Kraus W. Insulin resistance syndrome and cardiovascular disease: genetics and connections to skeletal muscle function. *Am Heart J* 1999;138:S413–6.

34. Hu FB, Sigal RJ, Rich-Edwards JW et al. Walking compared with vigorous physical activity and risk of type 2 diabetes in women: a prospective study. *JAMA* 1999;282:1433–9.

35. Knowler WC, Barrett-Connor E, Fowler SE et al. Reduction in the incidence of type 2 diabetes with lifestyle intervention or metformin. *N Engl J Med* 2002;346:393–403.

36. Tuomilehto J, Lindstrom J, Eriksson JG et al. Prevention of type 2 diabetes mellitus by changes in lifestyle among subjects with impaired glucose tolerance. *N Engl J Med* 2001;344:1343–50.

37. Wannamethee SG, Shaper AG, Alberti KG. Physical activity, metabolic factors, and the incidence of coronary heart disease and type 2 diabetes. *Arch Intern Med* 2000;160: 2108–16.

38. Kriska AM, Pereira MA, Hanson RL et al. Association of physical activity and serum insulin concentrations in two populations at high risk for type 2 diabetes but differing by BMI. *Diabetes Care* 2001;24:1175–80.

39. Hu FB, Leitzmann MF, Stampfer MJ et al. Physical activity and television watching in relation to risk for type 2 diabetes mellitus in men. *Arch Intern Med* 2001;161:1542–8.

40. Salmeron J, Ascherio A, Rimm EB et al. Dietary fiber, glycemic load, and risk of NIDDM in men. *Diabetes Care* 1997;20:545–50.

41. Meyer KA, Kushi LH, Jacobs DR Jr et al. Dietary fat and incidence of type 2 diabetes in older Iowa women. *Diabetes Care* 2001;24:1528–35.

42. van Dam RM, Rimm EB, Willett WC et al. Dietary patterns and risk for type 2 diabetes mellitus in US men. *Ann Intern Med* 2002;136:201–9.

43. Hu FB, Manson JE, Stampfer MJ et al. Diet, lifestyle, and the risk of type 2 diabetes mellitus in women. *N Engl J Med* 2001;345:790–7.

44. Liu S, Manson JE, Stampfer MJ et al. A prospective study of whole-grain intake and risk of type 2 diabetes mellitus in US women. *Am J Public Health* 2000;90:1409–15.

45. Eriksson KF, Lindgarde F. Prevention of type 2 (non-insulin-dependent) diabetes mellitus by diet and physical exercise. The 6-year Malmo feasibility study. *Diabetologia* 1991;34:891–8.

46. Pan XR, Li GW, Hu YH et al. Effects of diet and exercise in preventing NIDDM in people with impaired glucose tolerance. The Da Qing IGT and Diabetes Study. *Diabetes Care* 1997;20:537–44.

47. Chiasson JL, Josse RG, Gomis R et al. Acarbose for prevention of type 2 diabetes mellitus: the STOP-NIDDM randomised trial. *Lancet* 2002;359:2072–7.

48. Yusuf S, Gerstein H, Hoogwerf B et al. Ramipril and the development of diabetes. *JAMA* 2001;286:1882–5.

49. Hansson L, Lindholm LH, Niskanen L et al. Effect of angiotensin-converting-enzyme inhibition compared with conventional therapy on cardiovascular morbidity and mortality in hypertension: the Captopril Prevention Project (CAPPP) randomised trial. *Lancet* 1999;353:611–6.

50. Buchanan TA, Xiang AH, Peters RK et al. Preservation of pancreatic beta-cell function and prevention of type 2 diabetes by pharmacological treatment of insulin resistance in high-risk hispanic women. *Diabetes* 2002;51:2796–803.

51. Dahlof B, Devereux RB, Kjeldsen SE et al. Cardiovascular morbidity and mortality in the Losartan Intervention For Endpoint reduction in hypertension study (LIFE): a randomised trial against atenolol. *Lancet* 2002;359:995–1003.

52. American Diabetes Association. Role of cardiovascular risk factors in prevention and treatment of macrovascular disease in diabetes. *Diabetes Care* 1989;12:573–9.

53. Kannel WB, McGee DL. Diabetes and cardiovascular disease. The Framingham study. *JAMA* 1979;241:2035–8.

54. Wingard DL, Barrett-Connor E. Heart disease and diabetes. In: Harris M, ed. *Diabetes in America*. 2nd ed. Bethesda, MD: National Institute of Diabetes and Digestive and Kidney Diseases, 1995:429–48.

55. Geiss LS, Herman WH, Smith PJ. Mortality in non-insulin dependent diabetes. In: Harris M, ed. *Diabetes in America*. 2nd ed. Bethesda, MD: National Institute of Diabetes and Digestive and Kidney Diseases, 1995:233–55.

56. Stamler J, Vaccaro O, Neaton JD et al. Diabetes, other risk factors, and 12-yr cardiovascular mortality for men screened in the Multiple Risk Factor Intervention Trial. *Diabetes Care* 1993;16:434–44.

57. UK Prospective Diabetes Study (UKPDS) Group. Intensive blood-glucose control with sulphonylureas or insulin compared with conventional treatment and risk of complications in patients with type 2 diabetes (UKPDS 33). *Lancet* 1998;352:837–53.

58. Haffner SM, Lehto S, Ronnemaa T et al. Mortality from coronary heart disease in subjects with type 2 diabetes and in nondiabetic subjects with and without prior myocardial infarction. *N Engl J Med* 1998;339:229–34.

59. Aronson D, Rayfield EJ, Chesebro JH. Mechanisms determining course and outcome of diabetic patients who have had acute myocardial infarction. *Ann Intern Med* 1997;126:296–306.

60. McGuire DK, Emanuelsson H, Granger CB et al. Influence of diabetes mellitus on clinical outcomes across the spectrum of acute coronary syndromes. Findings from the GUSTO-IIb study. GUSTO IIb Investigators. *Eur Heart J* 2000;21:1750–8.

61. Malmberg K, Yusuf S, Gerstein HC et al. Impact of diabetes on long-term prognosis in patients with unstable angina and non-Q-wave myocardial infarction: results of the OASIS (Organization to Assess Strategies for Ischemic Syndromes) Registry. *Circulation* 2000;102:1014–9.

62. Gu K, Cowie CC, Harris MI. Mortality in adults with and without diabetes in a national cohort of the US population, 1971–1993. *Diabetes Care* 1998;21:1138–45.

63. Centers for Disease Control and Prevention. Major Cardiovascular Disease (CVD) During 1997–1999 and Major CVD Hospital Discharge Rates in 1997 Among Women with Diabetes — United States. *Morb Mortal Wkly Rep* 2001;50:948–54.

64. Fibrinolytic Therapy Trialists' (FTT) Collaborative Group. Indications for fibrinolytic therapy in suspected acute myocardial infarction: collaborative overview of early mortality and major morbidity results from all randomised trials of more than 1000 patients. *Lancet* 1994;343:311–22.

65. Granger CB, Califf RM, Young S et al. Outcome of patients with diabetes mellitus and acute myocardial infarction treated with thrombolytic agents. The Thrombolysis and Angioplasty in Myocardial Infarction (TAMI) Study Group. *J Am Coll Cardiol* 1993; 21:920–5.

66. Mak KH, Moliterno DJ, Granger CB et al. Influence of diabetes mellitus on clinical outcome in the thrombolytic era of acute myocardial infarction. GUSTO-I Investigators. Global Utilization of Streptokinase and Tissue Plasminogen Activator for Occluded Coronary Arteries. *J Am Coll Cardiol* 1997;30:171–9.

67. Abbott RD, Donahue RP, Kannel WB et al. The impact of diabetes on survival following myocardial infarction in men vs. women. The Framingham Study. *JAMA* 1988;260: 3456–60.

68. Kannel WB, Ho K, Thom T. Changing epidemiological features of cardiac failure. *Br Heart J* 1994;72 (Suppl. 2):S3–9.

69. Kannel WB, Hjortland M, Castelli WP. Role of diabetes in congestive heart failure: the Framingham study. *Am J Cardiol* 1974;34:29–34.

70. Dries DL, Sweitzer NK, Drazner MH et al. Prognostic impact of diabetes mellitus in patients with heart failure according to the etiology of left ventricular systolic dysfunction. *J Am Coll Cardiol* 2001;38:421–8.

71. Jaffe AS, Spadaro JJ, Schechtman K et al. Increased congestive heart failure after myocardial infarction of modest extent in patients with diabetes mellitus. *Am Heart J* 1984;108:31–7.

72. Stone PH, Muller JE, Hartwell T et al. The effect of diabetes mellitus on prognosis and serial left ventricular function after acute myocardial infarction: contribution of both coronary disease and diastolic left ventricular dysfunction to the adverse prognosis. The MILIS Study Group. *J Am Coll Cardiol* 1989;14:49–57.

73. Burchfiel CM, Curb JD, Rodriguez BL et al. Glucose intolerance and 22-year stroke incidence. The Honolulu Heart Program. *Stroke* 1994;25:951–7.

74. Palumbo PJ, Melton LJ. Peripheral vascular disease and diabetes. In: National Diabetes Group, ed. *Diabetes in America*. 2nd ed. Bethesda MD: National Institute of Diabetes and Digestive and Kidney Diseases, 1995:401–8.

75. Lanzer P. Topographic distribution of peripheral arteriopathy in non-diabetics and type 2 diabetics. *Z Kardiol* 2001;90:99–103.

76. Kreines K, Johnson E, Albrink M et al. The course of peripheral vascular disease in non-insulin-dependent diabetes. *Diabetes Care* 1985;8:235–43.

77. Niskanen L, Siitonen O, Suhonen M et al. Medial artery calcification predicts cardiovascular mortality in patients with NIDDM. *Diabetes Care* 1994;17:1252–6.

78. American Diabetes Association. Consensus Development Conference on Diabetic Foot Wound Care: 7–8 April 1999, Boston, Massachusetts. *Diabetes Care* 1999;22:1354–60.

79. Geiss LS, Rolka DB, Engelgau MM. Elevated blood pressure among US adults with diabetes, 1988–1994. *Am J Prev Med* 2002;22:42–8.

80. Klein R, Klein BE, Lee KE et al. The incidence of hypertension in insulin-dependent diabetes. *Arch Intern Med* 1996;156:622–7.

81. Reaven GM. Banting Lecture 1988: role of insulin resistance in human disease. *Diabetes* 1988;37:1595–607.

82. Bierman EL. George Lyman Duff Memorial Lecture. Atherogenesis in diabetes. *Arterioscler Thromb* 1992;12:647–56.

83. Garg A, Grundy SM. Diabetic dyslipidemia and its therapy. *Diabetes Review* 1997; 5:425–33.

84. Stampfer MJ, Krauss RM, Ma J et al. A prospective study of triglyceride level, low-density lipoprotein particle diameter, and risk of myocardial infarction. *JAMA* 1996;276:882–8.

85. Lamarche B, Tchernof A, Moorjani S et al. Small, dense low-density lipoprotein particles as a predictor of the risk of ischemic heart disease in men. Prospective results from the Quebec Cardiovascular Study. *Circulation* 1997;95:69–75.

86. Cowie CC, Harris MI. Physical and metabolic characteristics of persons with diabetes. In: National Diabetes Group, ed. *Diabetes in America*. 2nd ed. Bethesda MD: National Institute of Diabetes and Digestive and Kidney Diseases, 1995:117–64.

87. Gerstein HC, Pais P, Pogue J et al. Relationship of glucose and insulin levels to the risk of myocardial infarction: a case-control study. *J Am Coll Cardiol* 1999;33:612–9.

88. Kuusisto J, Mykkanen L, Pyorala K et al. NIDDM and its metabolic control predict coronary heart disease in elderly subjects. *Diabetes* 1994;43:960–7.

89. Singer DE, Nathan DM, Anderson KM et al. Association of HbA1c with prevalent cardiovascular disease in the original cohort of the Framingham Heart Study. *Diabetes* 1992;41:202–8.

90. Malmberg K, Norhammar A, Wedel H et al. Glycometabolic state at admission: important risk marker of mortality in conventionally treated patients with diabetes mellitus and acute myocardial infarction: long-term results from the Diabetes and Insulin-Glucose Infusion in Acute Myocardial Infarction (DIGAMI) study. *Circulation* 1999;99:2626–32.

91. Stern MP. The effect of glycemic control on the incidence of macrovascular complications of type 2 diabetes. *Arch Fam Med* 1998;7:155–62.

92. Meinert CL, Knatterud GL, Prout TE et al. A study of the effects of hypoglycemic agents on vascular complications in patients with adult-onset diabetes. II. Mortality results. *Diabetes* 1970;19 (Suppl.):789–830.

93. Abraira C, Colwell JA, Nuttall FQ et al. Veterans Affairs Cooperative Study on glycemic control and complications in type II diabetes (VA CSDM). Results of the feasibility trial. Veterans Affairs Cooperative Study in Type II Diabetes. *Diabetes Care* 1995;18:1113–23.

94. UK Prospective Diabetes Study (UKPDS) Group. Effect of intensive blood-glucose control with metformin on complications in overweight patients with type 2 diabetes (UKPDS 34). *Lancet* 1998;352:854–65.

95. Malmberg K, Ryden L, Efendic S et al. Randomized trial of insulin-glucose infusion followed by subcutaneous insulin treatment in diabetic patients with acute myocardial infarction (DIGAMI study): effects on mortality at 1 year. *J Am Coll Cardiol* 1995; 26:57–65.

96. Antiplatelet Trialist' Collaboration. Collaborative overview of randomised trials of antiplatelet therapy—I: prevention of death myocardial infarction and stroke by prolonged antiplatelet therapy in various categories of patients. *BMJ* 1994;308:81–106.

97. Steering Committee of the Physicians' Health Study Research Group. Final report on the aspirin component of the ongoing Physicians' Health Study. *N Engl J Med* 1989;321:129–35.

98. ETDRS Investigators. Aspirin effects on mortality and morbidity in patients with diabetes mellitus. Early Treatment Diabetic Retinopathy Study report 14. *JAMA* 1992;268:1292–300.

99. CAPRIE Steering Committee. A randomised, blinded, trial of clopidogrel versus aspirin in patients at risk of ischaemic events (CAPRIE). *Lancet* 1996;348:1329–39.

100. Yusuf S, Zhao F, Mehta SR et al. Effects of clopidogrel in addition to aspirin in patients with acute coronary syndromes without ST-segment elevation. *N Engl J Med* 2001; 345:494–502.

101. Nesto RW, Zarich S. Acute myocardial infarction in diabetes mellitus: lessons learned from ACE inhibition. *Circulation* 1998;97:12–5.

102. Yusuf S, Sleight P, Pogue J et al. Effects of an angiotensin-converting-enzyme inhibitor, ramipril, on cardiovascular events in high-risk patients. The Heart Outcomes Prevention Evaluation Study Investigators. *N Engl J Med* 2000;342:145–53.

103. Heart Outcomes Prevention Evaluation Study Investigators. Effects of ramipril on cardiovascular and microvascular outcomes in people with diabetes mellitus: results of the HOPE study and MICRO-HOPE substudy. *Lancet* 2000;355:253–9.

104. UK Prospective Diabetes Study Group. Tight blood pressure control and risk of macrovascular and microvascular complications in type 2 diabetes: UKPDS 38. *BMJ* 1998;317:703–13.

105. Curb JD, Pressel SL, Cutler JA et al. Effect of diuretic-based antihypertensive treatment on cardiovascular disease risk in older diabetic patients with isolated systolic hypertension. Systolic Hypertension in the Elderly Program Cooperative Research Group. *JAMA* 1996;276:1886–92.

106. Pyorala K, Pedersen TR, Kjekshus J et al. Cholesterol lowering with simvastatin improves prognosis of diabetic patients with coronary heart disease. A subgroup analysis of the Scandinavian Simvastatin Survival Study (4S). *Diabetes Care* 1997;20:614–20.

107. Sacks FM, Pfeffer MA, Moye LA et al. The effect of pravastatin on coronary events after myocardial infarction in patients with average cholesterol levels. Cholesterol and Recurrent Events Trial investigators. *N Engl J Med* 1996;335:1001–9.

108. The Long-term Intervention with Pravastatin in Ischaemic Disease (LIPID) Study Group. Prevention of cardiovascular events and death with pravastatin in patients with coronary heart disease and a broad range of initial cholesterol levels. The Long-Term Intervention with Pravastatin in Ischaemic Disease (LIPID) Study Group. *N Engl J Med* 1998;339:1349–57.

109. The Heart Protection Study Investigators. MRC/BHF Heart Protection Study of cholesterol lowering with simvastatin in 20,536 high-risk individuals: a randomised placebo-controlled trial. *Lancet* 2002;360:7–22.

110. American Diabetes Association. Standards of medical care for patients with diabetes mellitus. *Tenn Med* 2000;93:419–29.

111. Gibbons RJ, Chatterjee K, Daley J et al. ACC/AHA/ACP-ASIM guidelines for the management of patients with chronic stable angina: a report of the American College of Cardiology/American Heart Association Task Force on Practice Guidelines (Committee on Management of Patients With Chronic Stable Angina). *J Am Coll Cardiol* 1999; 33:2092–197.

112. Expert Panel on Detection and Treatment of High Blood Cholesterol in Adults. Executive Summary of the Third Report of the National Cholesterol Education Program (NCEP) Expert Panel on Detection, Evaluation, and Treatment of High Blood Cholesterol in Adults (Adult Treatment Panel III). *JAMA* 2001;285:2486–97.

113. The Joint National Committee on prevention, evaluation, and treatment of high blood pressure. The sixth report of the Joint National Committee on prevention, detection, evaluation, and treatment of high blood pressure. *Arch Intern Med* 1997;157:2413–46.

114. Lindholm LH, Ibsen H, Dahlof B et al. Cardiovascular morbidity and mortality in patients with diabetes in the Losartan Intervention For Endpoint reduction in hypertension study (LIFE): a randomised trial against atenolol. *Lancet* 2002; 359:1004–10.

115. The PURSUIT Trial Investigators. Inhibition of platelet glycoprotein IIb/IIIa with eptifibatide in patients with acute coronary syndromes. The PURSUIT Trial Investigators. Platelet Glycoprotein IIb/IIIa in Unstable Angina: Receptor Suppression Using Integrilin Therapy. *N Engl J Med* 1998;339:436–43.

116. The Platelet Receptor Inhibition in Ischemic Syndrome Management (PRISM) Study Investigators. A comparison of aspirin plus tirofiban with aspirin plus heparin for unstable angina. *N Engl J Med* 1998;338:1498–505.

117. The Platelet Receptor Inhibition in Ischemic Syndrome Management in Patients Limited by Unstable Angina Signs and Symptoms (PRISM-PLUS) Study Investigators. Inhibition of the platelet glycoprotein IIb/IIIa receptor with tirofiban in unstable angina and non-Q-wave myocardial infarction. *N Engl J Med* 1998;338:1488–97.

118. Roffi M, Chew DP, Mukherjee D et al. Platelet glycoprotein IIb/IIIa inhibitors reduce mortality in diabetic patients with non-ST-segment-elevation acute coronary syndromes. *Circulation* 2001;104:2767–71.

119. Bhatt DL, Marso SP, Lincoff AM et al. Abciximab reduces mortality in diabetics following percutaneous coronary intervention. *J Am Coll Cardiol* 2000;35:922–8.

120. Zimmet P, Alberti KG, Shaw J. Global and societal implications of the diabetes epidemic. *Nature* 2001;414:782–7.

121. Zimmet PZ, McCarty DJ, de Courten MP. The global epidemiology of non-insulin-dependent diabetes mellitus and the metabolic syndrome. *J Diabetes Complications* 1997;11:60–8.

122. Colditz GA, Willett WC, Rotnitzky A et al. Weight gain as a risk factor for clinical diabetes mellitus in women. *Ann Intern Med* 1995;122:481–6.

123. American Diabetes Association. Report of the Expert Committee on the Diagnosis and Classification of Diabetes Mellitus. *Diabetes Care* 1997;20:1183–97.

2

Pathophysiology

Steven P Marso

Introduction

The current pandemic of type 2 diabetes mellitus (T2DM) has emerged as a global health problem. There will soon be more than 200 million people with a history of diabetes mellitus worldwide. At present, there are 15.7 million diabetic people in the US, and conservative estimates suggest that one third of the US diabetic population remains undiagnosed. Over the next 20–30 years, the greatest health burden from T2DM will come from developing nations. Furthermore, an additional 40 million people in the US have insulin resistance syndrome and thus have a heightened risk for developing T2DM [1]. These numbers are projected to double over the next decade, with a disproportionate risk for developing T2DM among the elderly [2], children [3], and certain minority populations, including individuals of African and Hispanic origin.

Although the underpinnings of these epidemiologic observations have yet to be fully realized, there has been a parallel increase in the prevalence of societal obesity, sedentary lifestyles, and global "westernization" with respect to dietary preferences [4]. Unfortunately, cardiovascular complications remain the leading cause of death among patients with T2DM, accounting for 80% of all case fatalities. Although there has been a recent decline in age-adjusted mortality rates among patients with cardiovascular and cerebral vascular disease, there has not been a coinciding reduction in the age-adjusted mortality rates among patients with T2DM [5,6]. Although this paradox is not well understood, it underscores the pressing need for a continued pursuit of the key underlying biological mechanisms associated with T2DM and cardiovascular disease (CVD).

Patients with T2DM and CVD are clearly at an increased risk for intermediate and long-term adverse cardiovascular events, including, mortality following ST-segment elevation myocardial infarction (MI), acute coronary syndrome (ACS), coronary artery bypass grafting [7,8], and percutaneous coronary revascularization procedures [9,10]. For example, a recent meta-analysis that included data from six randomized controlled trials involving patients with an ACS demonstrated an odds ratio (OR) of nearly 2 for 30-day mortality among the diabetic cohort ($P < 0.001$) [11]. Similarly, a substudy analysis from TARGET (the do Tirofiban and ReoPro give Similar Efficacy Trial) clearly demonstrated that diabetic patients undergoing percutaneous coronary intervention (PCI) in the setting of an ACS remain at risk for 6-month adverse events including death, MI, or target vessel revascularization. Diabetic patients had an OR of 1.27 (95% confidence interval [CI]: 1.04–1.55, $P = 0.02$) for 6-month major adverse cardiac events (MACE) following multivariate analysis [12].

Figure 1 further stratifies the risk of in-hospital mortality based upon the high-risk clinical characteristics of diabetic patients undergoing PCI. There is almost a logarithmic increased risk for in-hospital death associated with the addition of the depicted clinical characteristics. In the modern day, there remains no question that people with diabetes are at increased risk for future cardiovascular events.

Pathogenesis of cardiovascular disease and T2DM

Numerous plausible biological mechanisms have been put forward to explain the early development of atherosclerosis and the exceptionally poor outcome of patients with T2DM and CVD. As well as aggressive atherosclerosis, patients with T2DM also exhibit:

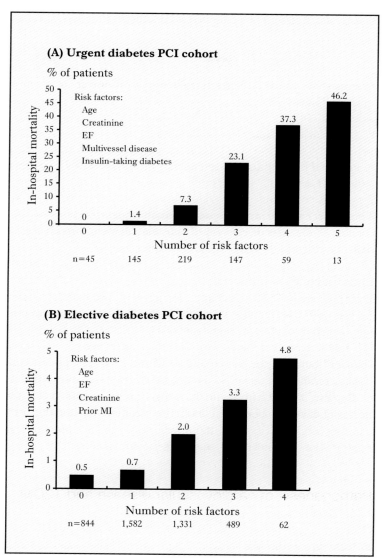

Figure 1. The increasing in-hospital mortality associated with depicted risk factors in: (**A**) an urgent diabetes percutaneous coronary intervention (PCI) cohort; and (**B**) an elective diabetes PCI cohort. EF: ejection fraction; MI: myocardial infarction.

- early development of an abnormal endothelial function

- platelet hyperactivity

- enhanced cellular and matrix proliferation following arterial injury

- a propensity for adverse arterial remodeling

- impaired fibrinolysis with a tendency for thrombosis and inflammation

These mechanisms are discussed in subsequent sections of this chapter. A detailed discussion of the tendency for thrombosis in patients with T2DM is provided in Chapter 3.

Endothelial dysfunction

Profound arteriopathy occurs during the prediabetic state. Endothelial dysfunction is perhaps the earliest demonstrable manifestation of this. A monolayer of endothelial cells (EC) lines the inner aspect of blood vessels. This layer serves as a vital "barrier" between the lumen and vessel wall tissue, and certainly plays a pivotal role in vessel homeostasis. Although the function of the EC layer continues to be actively investigated, biological functions that have been linked to normal endothelial function are:

- regulation of blood flow – including vasomotor tone

- hemostasis

- nutrient delivery

- leukocyte trafficking

- vascular smooth muscle cell proliferation and migration

Loss of normal endothelial cellular function is thought to be an early marker for the development of atherosclerosis, preceding the development of overt *de novo* atherosclerosis. T2DM leads to early endothelial injury, probably as a result of hyperglycemia, hypertension, diabetic dyslipidemia, and insulin resistance. Therefore, endothelial dysfunction is an early hallmark for the development of both micro- and macrovascular complications of T2DM.

Although vascular reactivity has been evaluated using several methods, endothelium-derived nitric oxide (NO) is usually the molecule that is monitored. Although, over 20 years ago, the description of NO resulted in a Nobel Prize for Furchgott, Ignarro, and Murad, the clinical implications for its biological activity – including EC-mediated flow dilation – remain to be further defined. Nonetheless, it does appear that diabetes significantly alters NO-mediated dilation, resulting in a propensity for vasoconstriction, inflammation, and thrombosis – ultimately culminating in atherosclerosis.

Impaired endothelial function is not only antecedent to the development of atherosclerosis, but is also demonstrable in the early stages of T2DM [13–15], and is likely to precede the onset of microalbuminuria [16]. Furthermore, individuals with impaired glucose tolerance (IGT) and first-degree relatives of patients with T2DM have a weakened response to acetylcholine, as measured by flow-mediated brachial artery diameter changes [17]. Additionally, patients with T2DM, first-degree relatives of patients with T2DM, and people with IGT have an increased circulating concentration of markers of endothelial dysfunction, including soluble vascular cell adhesion molecule (sVCAM), soluble intercellular adhesion molecule (sICAM), endothelin (ET)-1, and von Willebrand factor (vWF). These data support the notion that there is macrovascular risk well before the development of overt T2DM. Although there is clearly a clustering of cardiovascular risk factors prior to the development of T2DM, it remains likely that insulin resistance syndrome and/or the prediabetic state contribute to a substantial vascular risk beyond traditional risk factors.

The biological drivers of impaired endothelial function among subjects with T2DM are varied, but are undoubtedly linked to multiple NO pathways, including, diminished production of NO, increased inactivation by reactive oxygen species, and impaired signal transduction [18]. Hyperglycemia, whether via oxidant stress, diacylglycerol (DAG) production, or advanced glycation endproducts (AGEs), has been shown to activate protein kinase C (PKC) [19].

The PKC pathway has been well characterized and is associated with many abnormal cellular functions, including increased vascular contractility and endothelial dysfunction. It is likely that these functions are mediated via ET-1, angiotensin II, and endothelial NO synthase (eNOS). Although acute normalization of glucose levels does not translate into reduced levels of DAG or PKC activation in diabetic rat aortas [20], modulation of PKC via a specific inhibitor results in improved renal mesangial thickening, blood flow, and monocyte activation [21]. Furthermore, angiotensin-converting enzyme (ACE) inhibition has been shown to restore endothelium-dependent vasorelaxation in nonhypertensive type 1 [22] and type 2 patients [23].

It is also very likely that endothelial dysfunction is linked with circulating inflammatory cytokines [24]. Numerous epidemiological studies have linked an increase in the basal level of cytokines – such as interleukin (IL)-6 and C-reactive protein (CRP) [25,26] – to the development of both T2DM and central adiposity. Recent studies have demonstrated that modulating the cytokine axis – either with pharmacologic agents [27] or a reduction in visceral fat [28] – results in a net improvement in endothelial function and a reduction in the circulating levels of cytokines and soluble markers of EC activation [28].

Clinical assessment of endothelial function

Although no gold standard exists for the clinical quantification of endothelial function, several modalities are utilized to quantify vascular reactivity. Initially, acetylcholine in the human coronary circulation was used to assess endothelium-dependent relaxation [29]. Endothelial function is determined invasively using quantitative coronary angiography or a Doppler flow wire. With quantitative coronary angiography, the epicardial lumen diameter is measured following the administration of an endothelium-dependent vasodilator, such as acetylcholine or serotonin. The Doppler flow wire assesses microvascular endothelial function by measuring the coronary flow reserve.

The major limitation with these modalities is the requirement for invasive cannulation of coronary arteries. Consequently, minimally invasive strategies to assess endothelial function have been developed. One such technique employs high-resolution ultrasound to measure flow-mediated dilation (FMD) and is dependent upon hyperemic-mediated dilation of the brachial artery. This method was first applied clinically in the early 1990s [30], and further studies over the last decade have indicated an acceptable reliability for the measurement of FMD [30–35]. In this model, the artery of interest – usually the brachial or superficial femoral artery – is occluded using a cuff inflation protocol for 4–5 minutes. The diameter of the target artery is then measured, at rest and following hyperemia, using 2-dimensional ultrasound images. This model appears to be an adequate method for the noninvasive detection of endothelial function and has been demonstrated to be useful in disease states such as hypertension [33], T2DM [36], and among persons at risk for coronary artery disease (CAD) [37].

Another noninvasive tool to assess endothelial function is venous plethysmography. In this model, forearm blood flow (FBF) is measured as originally described by Hokanson and coworkers in 1975 [38]. This technique has shown that although basal FBF appears similar among people with and without diabetes, the vasodilative response is attenuated among diabetic subjects compared with controls [39,40]. Other tools to clinically evaluate the endothelium include a measurement of intimal medial thickness, pulse wave velocity, and positron emission tomography [41].

Platelet hyperactivity

The diabetic platelet has emerged as a distinct target for therapeutic intervention. Increased platelet activity is certainly involved in the increased thrombogenic potential among diabetic patients. Diabetic platelets are larger, have a greater number of glycoprotein (GP)IIb/IIIa receptors [42], and aggregate more readily to known agonists *in vitro* than platelets from nondiabetic patients [43].

Knobler et al. compared shear-induced whole-blood platelet adhesion and aggregation on subendothelial extracellular matrix between diabetic and nondiabetic patients. This *ex vivo* model closely approximates the *in vivo* environment by maintaining all other blood elements, shear force, and solid-phase subendothelial components [44]. The study demonstrated increased platelet adhesion and aggregation in diabetic patients, loosely correlating with the degree of dyslipidemia. Furthermore, a greater percentage of diabetic platelets circulate in an activated state, which may be caused by an increased production of F2-isoprostane due to hyperglycemia [45]. Also, serum glucose may promote platelet-mediated thrombosis.

Sheachter et al. demonstrated that serum glucose levels were a key multivariate predictor of platelet-dependent thrombosis (PDT) [46]. In this study, serum glucose, apolipoprotein B (APOB), and intracellular magnesium correlated with PDT among patients with stable CAD.

Table 1 depicts the many abnormalities in the pathobiology of platelet aggregation among patients with T2DM. Prostacyclin (PGI$_2$) and NO are two well-characterized molecules with potent

Characteristic	Insulin resistance	T2DM
Insulin-mediated antiaggregation	↓	↓
NO-mediated antiaggregation	↓	↓
Prostacyclin-mediated antiaggregation	↓	↓
cGMP response to NO	↓	↓
cNOS activity	→	↓
iNOS activity	→	↑
Thrombin-induced PI hydrolysis	→	↑
Thromboxane synthesis	→	↑

Table 1. Platelet dysfunction in insulin resistant and type 2 diabetic patients (T2DM). cGMP: cyclic guanosine monophosphate; cNOS: constitutive nitric oxide synthase; iNOS: inducible nitric oxide synthase; NO: nitric oxide; PAI-1: plasminogen activator inhibitor-1; PI: phosphoinositide; ↑: increased; ↓: decreased; →: no change. Adapted with permission from Vinik AI, Erbas T, Park TS et al. Platelet dysfunction in type 2 diabetes. *Diabetes Care* 2001:24;1476–85.

antiplatelet aggregation properties. These compounds are released by intact vascular endothelium and inhibit the effects of numerous proaggregating agents. A decrease in the antiaggregatory activity of both PGI_2 and NO may well play a pivotal role in the pathobiology of platelet function in T2DM. Additionally, the synthesis of platelet-derived proaggregatory substances – such as ADP and thromboxane A_2 – is upregulated in patients with diabetes and insulin resistance. This results in a propensity for platelet-mediated atherothrombosis among T2DM patients.

Given the aforementioned abnormalities in platelet function, it is not surprising that T2DM patients derive marked clinical benefit from an antiplatelet treatment strategy. Many studies have convincingly shown improved cardiovascular outcomes with a range of antiplatelet agents, including aspirin [47–49], thienopyridine derivatives such as clopidogrel [50], and the GPIIb/IIIa receptor inhibitors. The GPIIb/IIIa receptor binds fibrinogen, resulting in platelet crosslinking, and is obligatory for the process of platelet aggregation. Modulation of the GPIIb/IIIa axis among patients with T2DM presenting with an ACS and/or PCI has resulted in improved short- and long-term event-free survival among diabetic patients.

The early safety and long-term efficacy of the first GPIIb/IIIa receptor antagonist developed – abciximab – has been extensively evaluated among patients with T2DM undergoing PCI, who have consistently been shown to be at heightened risk following PCI [51]. The addition of abciximab to the treatment strategy improved the early safety and long-term efficacy of percutaneous coronary revascularization in diabetic patients.

These initial findings have been further substantiated by a pooled analysis from the EPIC (Evaluation of c7E3 for the Prevention of Ischemic Complications), EPILOG (Evaluation of PTCA [percutaneous transluminal coronary angioplasty] to Improve Long-term Outcome with Abciximab GPIIb/IIIa Blockade), and EPISTENT (Evaluation of Platelet IIb/IIIa Inhibitor for Stenting Trial) trials involving PCI patients [52]. In this meta-analysis, there was nearly a 50% reduction in 1-year mortality for those diabetic patients receiving abciximab at the time of PCI (4.5% vs. 2.5%, $P = 0.031$). The efficacy of abciximab persisted among high-risk subgroups of diabetic patients, including those with clinical markers of insulin resistance (5.1% vs. 2.3% $P = 0.0044$), insulin-requiring diabetic patients (8.1% vs. 4.2%, $P = 0.073$), and those diabetic patients undergoing multivessel intervention (7.7% vs. 0.9%, $P = 0.018$). A meta-analysis by Roffi extended the understanding of GPIIb/IIIa inhibition among diabetic patients to the setting of ACS by demonstrating a marked reduction in mortality in patients who received an intravenous GPIIb/IIIa inhibitor, regardless of the revascularization strategy [11].

Cellular proliferation and matrix deposition

It has consistently been shown that T2DM patients have higher rates of restenosis following PCI. This was first noted in a report from the National Heart, Lung, and Blood Institute, which summarized the early balloon angioplasty experience [53]. Since then, several other studies have confirmed the conclusions of this report.

Restenosis following balloon arterial dilation is a result of abrupt vessel closure, adverse arterial remodeling, and proliferation of neointima. The advent of stenting has resulted in improved vessel patency rates due to a reduction in the incidence of restenosis in diabetic and nondiabetic patients. This reduction is primarily caused by the elimination of abrupt closure and vessel remodeling following PCI. Restenosis following stenting is a direct result of neointimal proliferation. Patients with T2DM continue to have higher rates of restenosis than nondiabetic patients following both balloon angioplasty and stenting.

Both insulin and glucose have been implicated as the key drivers of neointimal proliferation among patients with T2DM. Hyperglycemia affects many growth factors, including basic fibroblast growth factor and transforming growth factor-α [54]. Additionally, the synthesis of matrix components – such as collagen type IV, fibronectin, and laminin – is increased with hyperglycemia [55]. Hyperglycemia also results in diminished production of heparin sulfate, which allows a greater reduction in inhibition of cellular proliferation [56]. This may further promote expansion of the neointima following arterial injury. Also, hyperglycemia leads to the formation of AGEs, which induce inflammatory cell recruitment and cellular proliferation. Modulation of AGEs and the receptor for the AGE axis results in a significant reduction in the area of neointima proliferation in an insulin-resistant Zucker rat restenosis model [57].

It is unlikely that hyperglycemia is the sole key modulator of restenosis among T2DM patients. Many animal models and human

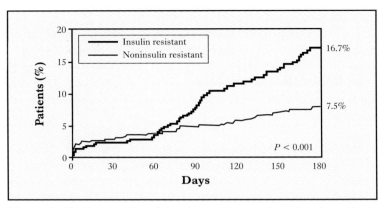

Figure 2. The 1-year rates of target vessel revascularization for patients enrolled in EPISTENT. The two groups depicted are those with the triad of diabetes mellitus, hypertension, and obesity.

studies of restenosis have failed to clearly link glucose to restenosis following arterial injury. Although insulin is a weak growth factor [58], the coexpression of insulin-like growth factor-1 and platelet-derived growth factor has a potent mitogenic effect and may play a role in the multifaceted process of restenosis.

Although the key biological drivers are not yet known, insulin resistance has been associated with restenosis. A small human study suggested that insulin resistance – as measured by the area under the curve for insulin production following an oral glucose tolerance test – was associated with an increased risk of restenosis following PCI [59]. Animal restenosis models have suggested that insulin resistance, rather than an insulin-deficient state, promotes extracellular deposition following arterial injury. In further support of this, clinical markers of insulin resistance, including hypertension, obesity, and diabetes, were associated with an increased risk of 1-year target vessel revascularization in EPISTENT (see **Figure 2**) [51].

These observations have led to a formal prospective evaluation of insulin resistance utilizing homeostasis model assessment

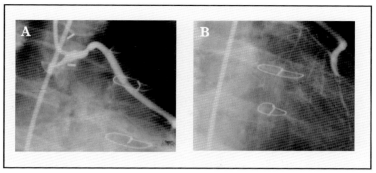

Figure 3. (A,B) Angiographic pictures of a saphenous venous graft to a diffusely diseased left anterior descending artery in a patient with type 2 diabetes.

(HOMA) among nondiabetic patients within the CREDO (Clopidogrel for Reduction of Events During Observation) insulin resistance substudy. The main objective of this substudy was to determine if insulin resistance was associated with an increased rate of 1-year target vessel revascularization.

Adverse arterial remodeling

Diabetes mellitus affects approximately 8%–10% of the world population. However, around 15%–25% of persons presenting with an ACS or those undergoing a coronary revascularization procedure have a history of diabetes mellitus. In addition to a propensity for vessel renarrowing following arterial injury, patients with diabetes have many other abnormal vessel properties that place them at risk for future cardiovascular events. Patients with diabetes exhibit aggressive atherosclerosis (see **Figure 3**), including, a tendency for negative arterial remodeling during the early stages of atherosclerosis, lack of collateral vessel formation, and a heightened risk of late vessel occlusion following conventional balloon angioplasty (i.e., prior to the advent of intracoronary stenting).

Fifteen years ago, Glagov and colleagues demonstrated an early compensatory arterial dilation in the presence of initial *de novo* atherosclerosis in the left main trunk of human cadaveric subjects

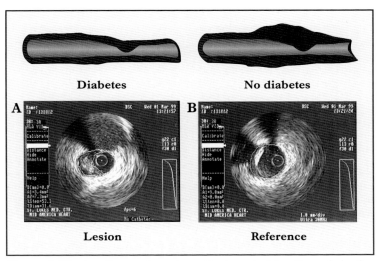

Figure 4. The top diagram is a schematic characterizing the maladaptive arterial remodeling process thought to occur in patients with diabetes mellitus. This concept is demonstrated in two representative intravascular ultrasound pictures from: (**A**) a diseased portion of the ostial left anterior descending artery; and (**B**) a "normal distal" reference from the mid-left anterior descending artery.

[60]. Compensatory dilation of the internal elastic lamina was observed in the presence of atherosclerotic disease, thus maintaining a "normal" luminal area for plaque areas up to 40%. Unfortunately, it has been shown that patients with diabetes exhibit a maladaptive arterial remodeling process (see **Figure 4**).

Instead of having an adaptive arterial response to the development of atherosclerosis, patients with diabetes exhibit vessel contracture, resulting in significant luminal stenosis with less plaque mass than in nondiabetic patients [61]. The intravascular ultrasound shown in **Figure 4A** is a still-frame image from the ostial portion of the left anterior descending artery. The vessel area – including an approximate 50% stenosis – is 7.2 mm^2 (see **Figure 4B**). The distal reference has a vessel area of approximately 9.0 mm^2. Due to this maladaptive remodeling process, arteries of diabetic patients are

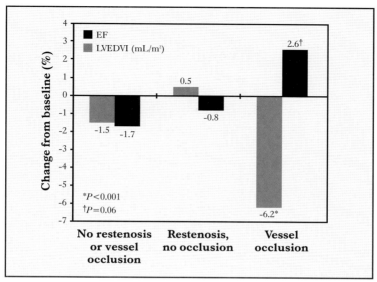

Figure 5. Bar graph depicting the changes in left ventricular remodeling and function in patients with occlusive restenosis. EF: ejection fraction; LVEDVI: left ventricular end-diastolic volume index. Adapted with permission from Physician's health study: aspirin and primary prevention of coronary heart disease. *N Engl J Med* 1989;321:1825–8.

often smaller, have longer lesion lengths, and are diffusely diseased. These morphological features also lead to an increased rate of intermediate and long-term complications following PCI.

The "typical" diabetic arteriopathy following balloon angioplasty results in a higher than expected rate of late-vessel occlusion. Studies conducted by Van Belle and colleagues have shown that patients with diabetes mellitus have late-vessel occlusion rates approximating 15% following balloon angioplasty. This number is markedly higher than the 3%–4% rate of occlusion following angioplasty that was previously reported [62]. Among this cohort, late-vessel occlusion resulted in adverse left ventricular remodeling (see **Figure 5**). Studies also showed that patients with occlusive restenosis had a significantly higher risk of 10-year cardiovascular mortality.

Although patients with diabetes have a propensity for both an aggressive form and an early onset of coronary atherosclerosis, diabetic patients seem to be less likely to collateralize severely diseased or occluded arterial segments [63]. The biological drivers for collateral vessel formation are likely to be complex, but preliminary work suggests a decreased gene expression of vascular endothelial growth factor (VEGF) in diabetic human myocardial samples. As expected in this study, there was a significant increase in VEGF mRNA expression in nondiabetic patients with documented CAD compared with controls. Patients with diabetes actually had decreased levels of VEGF expression compared with controls, as well as a decrease in expression of the VEGF receptor. Regardless of the underlying pathogenesis, there does appear to be a decrease in arteriogenesis among patients with T2DM and CAD.

Conclusion

Patients with diabetes provide unique challenges for both the clinical and scientific communities. Given the aggressive nature of coronary atherosclerosis, the differential response to mechanical revascularization, and the relatively poor cardiovascular event-free survival rate, efforts must continue to ensure an enlightened medical community, an informed public, and adequate resources to care for this ever-increasing population.

References

1. Ford ES, Giles WH, Dietz WH. Prevalence of the metabolic syndrome among US adults: findings from the third National Health and Nutrition Examination Survey. *JAMA* 2002;287:356–9.
2. Winegard DL, Barrett-Connor E. Heart Disease and Diabetes. In: Harris MI, ed. *Diabetes in America*. 2nd ed. Bethesda, MD: National Institute of Diabetes and Digestion and Kidney Diseases, 1995:429–48.
3. Fagot-Campagna A. Emergence of type 2 diabetes mellitus in children: epidemiological evidence. *J Pediatr Endocrinol Metab* 2000;13 (Suppl. 6):1395–402.
4. Harris MI. Diabetes in America: epidemiology and scope of the problem. *Diabetes Care* 1998;21(Suppl. 3):C11–4.
5. McKinlay J, Marceau L. US public health and the 21st century: diabetes mellitus. *Lancet* 2000;356:757–61.
6. Gu K, Cowie CC, Harris MI. Diabetes and decline in heart disease mortality in US adults. *JAMA* 1999;281:1291–7.

7. Serruys PW, Costa MA, Betriu A et al. The influence of diabetes mellitus on clinical outcome following multivessel stenting or CABG in the ARTS trial. Circulation 1999;100 (Suppl. 1):1–364.

8. Marso SP, Ellis SG, Gurm HS et al. Proteinuria is a key determinant of death in patients with diabetes after isolated coronary artery bypass grafting. *Am Heart J* 2000;139:939–44.

9. Marso SP, Ellis SG, Tuzcu M et al. The importance of proteinuria as a determinant of mortality following percutaneous coronary revascularization in diabetics. *J Am Coll Cardiol* 1999;33:1269–77.

10. Kip KE, Faxon DP, Detre KM et al. Coronary angioplasty in diabetic patients. The National Heart, Lung, and Blood Institute Percutaneous Transluminal Coronary Angioplasty Registry. *Circulation* 1996;94:1818–25.

11. Roffi M, Chew DP, Mukherjee D et al. Platelet glycoprotein IIb/IIIa inhibitors reduce mortality in diabetic patients with non-ST-segment-elevation acute coronary syndromes. *Circulation* 2001;104:2767–71.

12. Stone GW, Moliterno DJ, Bertrand M et al. Impact of clinical syndrome acuity on the differential response to 2 glycoprotein IIb/IIIa inhibitors in patients undergoing coronary stenting: the TARGET Trial. *Circulation* 2002;105:2347–54.

13. Williams SB, Cusco JA, Roddy MA et al. Impaired nitric oxide-mediated vasodilation in patients with non-insulin-dependent diabetes mellitus. *J Am Coll Cardiol* 1996;27: 567–74.

14. McVeigh GE, Brennan GM, Johnston GD et al. Impaired endothelium-dependent and independent vasodilation in patients with type 2 (non-insulin-dependent) diabetes mellitus. *Diabetologia* 1992;35:771–6.

15. Morris SJ, Shore AC, Tooke JE. Responses of the skin microcirculation to acetylcholine and sodium nitroprusside in patients with NIDDM. *Diabetologia* 1995;38:1337–44.

16. Lim SC, Caballero AE, Smakowski P et al. Soluble intercellular adhesion molecule, vascular cell adhesion molecule, and impaired microvascular reactivity are early markers of vasculopathy in type 2 diabetic individuals without microalbuminuria. *Diabetes Care* 1999;22:1865–70.

17. Saito Y, Nakao K, Mukoyama M et al. Increased plasma endothelin level in patients with essential hypertension. *N Engl J Med* 1990;322:205.

18. Pilote L, Miller DP, Califf RM et al. Determinants of the use of coronary angiography and revascularization after thrombolysis for acute myocardial infarction. *N Engl J Med* 1996;335:1198–205.

19. Naruse K, King G. Effect of diabetes on endothelial function. In: Veves A, ed. *Diabetes and cardiovascular disease*. Totowa: Humana Press Inc., 2001:45–64.

20. Inoguchi T, Battan R, Handler E et al. Preferential elevation of protein kinase C isoform beta II and diacylglycerol levels in the aorta and heart of diabetic rats: differential reversibility to glycemic control by islet cell transplantation. *Proc Natl Acad Sci USA* 1992;89:11059–63.

21. Ishii H, Jirousek MR, Koya D et al. Amelioration of vascular dysfunctions in diabetic rats by an oral PKC beta inhibitor. *Science* 1996;272:728–31.

22. Arcaro G, Zenere BM, Saggiani F et al. ACE inhibitors improve endothelial function in type 1 diabetic patients with normal arterial pressure and microalbuminuria. *Diabetes Care* 1999;22:1536–42.

23. O'Driscoll G, Green D, Maiorana A et al. Improvement in endothelial function by angiotensin-converting enzyme inhibition in non-insulin-dependent diabetes mellitus. *J Am Coll Cardiol* 1999;33:1506–11.

24. Tomai F, Crea F, Gaspardone A et al. Unstable angina and elevated C-reactive protein levels predict enhanced vasoreactivity of the culprit lesion. *Circulation* 2001;104:1471–6.

25. Pradhan AD, Manson JE, Rifai N et al. C-reactive protein, interleukin 6, and risk of developing type 2 diabetes mellitus. *JAMA* 2001;286:327–34.

26. Festa A, D'Agostino R Jr, Howard G et al. Chronic subclinical inflammation as part of the insulin resistance syndrome: the Insulin Resistance Atherosclerosis Study (IRAS). *Circulation* 2000;102:42–7.

27. Fichtlscherer S, Rosenberger G, Walter DH et al. Elevated C-reactive protein levels and impaired endothelial vasoreactivity in patients with coronary artery disease. *Circulation* 2000;102:1000–6.

28. Ziccardi P, Nappo F, Giugliano G et al. Reduction of inflammatory cytokine concentrations and improvement of endothelial functions in obese women after weight loss over one year. *Circulation* 2002;105:804–9.

29. Ludmer PL, Selwyn AP, Shook TL et al. Paradoxical vasoconstriction induced by acetylcholine in atherosclerotic coronary arteries. *N Engl J Med* 1986;315:1046–51.

30. Celermajer DS, Sorensen KE, Gooch VM et al. Non-invasive detection of endothelial dysfunction in children and adults at risk of atherosclerosis. *Lancet* 1992;340:1111–5.

31. Corretti MC, Plotnick GD, Vogel RA. Technical aspects of evaluating brachial artery vasodilatation using high-frequency ultrasound. *Am J Physiol* 1995;268:H1397–404.

32. Celermajer DS, Sorensen KE, Georgakopoulos D et al. Cigarette smoking is associated with dose-related and potentially reversible impairment of endothelium-dependent dilation in healthy young adults. *Circulation* 1993;88:2149–55.

33. Li J, Zhao SP, Li XP et al. Non-invasive detection of endothelial dysfunction in patients with essential hypertension. *Int J Cardiol* 1997;61:165–9.

34. Enderle MD, Schroeder S, Ossen R et al. Comparison of peripheral endothelial dysfunction and intimal media thickness in patients with suspected coronary artery disease. *Heart* 1998;80:349–54.

35. Anderson TJ, Uehata A, Gerhard MD et al. Close relation of endothelial function in the human coronary and peripheral circulations. *J Am Coll Cardiol* 1995;26:1235–41.

36. Veves A, Saouaf R, Donaghue VM et al. Aerobic exercise capacity remains normal despite impaired endothelial function in the micro- and macrocirculation of physically active IDDM patients. *Diabetes* 1997;46:1846–52.

37. Clarkson P, Celermajer DS, Powe AJ et al. Endothelium-dependent dilatation is impaired in young healthy subjects with a family history of premature coronary disease. *Circulation* 1997;96:3378–83.

38. Hokanson DE, Sumner DS, Strandness DE Jr. An electrically calibrated plethysmograph for direct measurement of limb blood flow. *IEEE Trans Biomed Eng* 1975;22:25–9.

39. Johnstone MT, Creager SJ, Scales KM et al. Impaired endothelium-dependent vasodilation in patients with insulin-dependent diabetes mellitus. *Circulation* 1993;88:2510–6.

40. Smits P, Kapma JA, Jacobs MC et al. Endothelium-dependent vascular relaxation in patients with type I diabetes. *Diabetes* 1993;42:148–53.

41. Beanlands RS, Muzik O, Melon P et al. Noninvasive quantification of regional myocardial flow reserve in patients with coronary atherosclerosis using nitrogen-13 ammonia positron emission tomography. Determination of extent of altered vascular reactivity. *J Am Coll Cardiol* 1995;26:1465–75.

42. Tschoepe D, Roesen P, Kaufmann L et al. Evidence for abnormal platelet glycoprotein expression in diabetes mellitus. *Eur J Clin Invest* 1990;20:166–70.

43. Aronson D, Bloomgarden Z, Rayfield EJ. Potential mechanisms promoting restenosis in diabetic patients. *J Am Coll Cardiol* 1996;27:528–35.

44. Knobler H, Savion N, Shenkman B et al. Shear-induced platelet adhesion and aggregation on subendothelium are increased in diabetic patients. *Thromb Res* 1998;90:181–90.

45. Davi G, Ciabattoni G, Consoli A et al. *In vivo* formation of 8-iso-prostaglandin f2alpha and platelet activation in diabetes mellitus: effects of improved metabolic control and vitamin E supplementation. *Circulation* 1999;99:224–9.

46. Shechter M, Merz CN, Paul-Labrador MJ et al. Blood glucose and platelet-dependent thrombosis in patients with coronary artery disease. *J Am Coll Cardiol* 2000;35:300–7.

47. Collaborative overview of randomised trials of antiplatelet therapy—I: Prevention of death, myocardial infarction, and stroke by prolonged antiplatelet therapy in various categories of patients. Anti-platelet Trialists' Collaboration. *BMJ* 1994;308:81–106.

48. Physician's health study: aspirin and primary prevention of coronary heart disease. *N Engl J Med* 1989;321:1825–8.

49. Aspirin effects on mortality and morbidity in patients with diabetes mellitus. Early Treatment Diabetic Retinopathy Study report 14. ETDRS Investigators. *JAMA* 1992;268:1292–300.

50. Bhatt DL, Marso SP, Hirsch AT et al. Superiority of clopidogrel versus aspirin in patients with a history of diabetes mellitus. *J Am Coll Cardiol* 2000;35:409A.

51. Marso SP, Lincoff AM, Ellis SG et al. Optimizing the percutaneous interventional outcomes for patients with diabetes mellitus: results of the EPISTENT (Evaluation of Platelet IIb/IIIa Inhibitor for Stenting Trial) diabetic substudy. *Circulation* 1999;100:2477–84.

52. Bhatt DL, Marso SP, Lincoff AM et al. Abciximab reduces mortality in diabetics following percutaneous coronary intervention. *J Am Coll Cardiol* 2000;35:922–8.

53. Holmes DR Jr, Vlietstra RE, Smith HC et al. Restenosis after percutaneous transluminal coronary angioplasty (PTCA): a report from the PTCA Registry of the National Heart, Lung, and Blood Institute. *Am J Cardiol* 1984;53:77–81C.

54. McClain DA, Paterson AJ, Roos MD et al. Glucose and glucosamine regulate growth factor gene expression in vascular smooth muscle cells. *Proc Natl Acad Sci USA* 1992;89:8150–4.

55. Roy S, Sala R, Cagliero E et al. Overexpression of fibronectin induced by diabetes or high glucose: phenomenon with a memory. *Proc Natl Acad Sci USA* 1990;87:404–8.

56. Unger E, Pettersson I, Eriksson UJ et al. Decreased activity of the heparan sulfate-modifying enzyme glucosaminyl N-deacetylase in hepatocytes from streptozotocin-diabetic rats. *J Biol Chem* 1991;266:8671–4.

57. Zhou ZM, Marso SP, Schmidt AM et al. Blockade of receptor for advanced glycation end-products (RAGE) suppresses neointimal formation in diabetic rat carotid artery injury model. *Circulation* 2000;102:(Suppl. II):246.

58. Bornfeldt KE, Raines EW, Nakano T et al. Insulin-like growth factor-I and platelet-derived growth factor-BB induce directed migration of human arterial smooth muscle cells via signaling pathways that are distinct from those of proliferation. *J Clin Invest* 1994;93:1266–74.

59. Nishimoto Y, Miyazaki Y, Toki Y et al. Enhanced secretion of insulin plays a role in the development of atherosclerosis and restenosis of coronary arteries: elective percutaneous transluminal coronary angioplasty in patients with effort angina. *J Am Coll Cardiol* 1998;32:1624–9.

60. Glagov S, Weisenberg E, Zarins CK et al. Compensatory enlargement of human atherosclerotic coronary arteries. *N Engl J Med* 1987;316:1371–5.

61. Kornowski R, Mintz GS, Lansky AJ et al. Paradoxic decreases in atherosclerotic plaque mass in insulin-treated diabetic patients. *Am J Cardiol* 1998;81:1298–304.

62. Van Belle E, Abolmaali K, Bauters C et al. Restenosis, late vessel occlusion and left ventricular function six months after balloon angioplasty in diabetic patients. *J Am Coll Cardiol* 1999;34:476–85.

63. Abaci A, Oguzhan A, Kahraman S et al. Effect of diabetes mellitus on formation of coronary collateral vessels. *Circulation* 1999;99:2239–42.

3

Hemostasis

Robert AS Ariëns & Peter J Grant

Introduction

Hemostasis is the term used to indicate the processes associated with the arrest of blood flow. These processes are usually triggered by external (wounding) or internal (atherosclerotic plaque rupture) injury to a blood vessel. Numerous cellular and enzymatic interactions are involved in the process, such as: platelet aggregation to form a primary hemostatic plug; a sequence of specific serine protease zymogen-to-enzyme conversions leading to the deposition of fibrin; and a counteracting enzymatic system of fibrinolysis to dissolve the fibrin–platelet plug.

The hemostatic equilibrium is determined by genetic, environmental, and metabolic factors; imbalances lead to bleeding or thrombosis. This chapter provides an up-to-date overview of the biological processes associated with hemostasis, followed by a discussion of the relationship between alterations in this system and the risk for micro- and macrovascular thrombotic disorders in patients with diabetes.

Biochemistry of coagulation

The coagulation cascade plays a central role in hemostasis. Specific zymogen-to-enzyme conversions lead to the formation of thrombin, which activates and aggregates platelets, converts fibrinogen to fibrin, and activates mechanisms that feed back positively or negatively on the system.

Trigger

Traditionally the coagulation cascade has been divided into two pathways, the intrinsic and extrinsic pathways; each pathway is triggered by a different mechanism. In 1964, the "waterfall" and "cascade" theories were proposed for the intrinsic pathway of coagulation [1,2]. The intrinsic pathway is triggered by activation of factor XII (see **Figure 1**). The extrinsic pathway of coagulation is triggered by tissue factor (TF). Although it has been known since the 19th century that the brain and other tissues contain a factor that induces blood clotting, it was not until the discovery that TF acts as a cofactor for factor VII in 1966 that the extrinsic pathway was characterized (see **Figure 1**) [3].

Intrinsic pathway activation

The classical dogma states that TF and negatively charged surfaces, such as glass, trigger coagulation independently. This theory has since been replaced by the current consensus that the main trigger for coagulation upon injury *in vivo* is TF [4]. Some researchers have expressed the view that contact activation of the intrinsic pathway could be a laboratory artifact, with activation only occurring when blood comes into contact with glass tubes. However, there are circumstances where contact activation plays a role in triggering coagulation *in vivo*, such as during extracorporeal circulation when the blood is exposed to negatively charged surfaces in the apparatus, although even in this situation contact activation does not always occur [5,6]. In addition, contact activation plays an important role in linking the activation of the coagulation, fibrinolysis, complement, and kinin pathways during thrombosis and sepsis (see **Figure 2**) [7].

Extrinsic pathway activation

TF is abundantly expressed on cells that surround the blood vessel; the brain, lungs, and placenta are particularly rich in TF. The perivascular distribution of TF ensures that clotting is readily triggered when the vasculature is injured, allowing blood to react with TF-rich cells. Intravascular cells – such as monocytes and endothelial cells – are also capable of expressing TF when stimulated by cytokines [8]. In addition, functionally active TF has

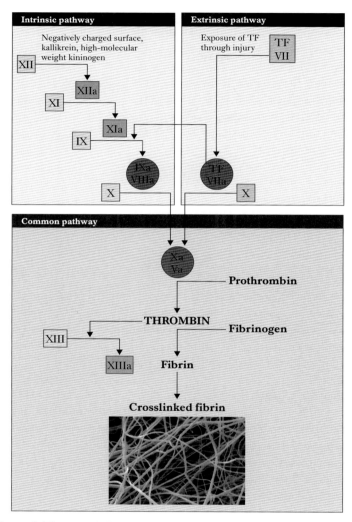

Figure 1. The coagulation cascade. Coagulation leads to the formation of a crosslinked fibrin clot. Vitamin K-dependent enzyme complexes (IXa/VIIIa, TF/VIIa, and Xa/Va) that require calcium and negatively charged phospholipids for full enzymatic activity are circled. Thrombin plays a central role in hemostasis, not only converting fibrinogen into fibrin and activating factor XIII, but also activating platelets and factors V, VIII, and XI. TF: tissue factor.

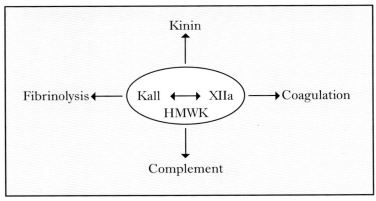

Figure 2. The reciprocal activation of factor XIIa and kallikrein (Kall) in the presence of high-molecular weight kininogen (HMWK) plays a linking role between the activation of the coagulation, complement, fibrinolysis, and kinin pathways.

been localized in the lipid-rich core of the atherosclerotic plaque, especially in association with macrophage-derived foam cells [9]. Intravascular expression of functionally active TF is kept under control by circulating TF pathway inhibitor (TFPI), which forms a complex with activated factor Xa, TF, and factor VIIa [10].

Studies have shown the existence of a pool of circulating or "blood-borne" TF [11]. Circulating TF propagates thrombus formation [12], but it is not known currently if it also plays a role in triggering coagulation. It has been suggested that circulating TF may be shed by microparticles from monocytes or polymorphonuclear leukocytes; however, a definite source has yet to be identified.

Cascade of zymogen-to-enzyme conversions

Factor VIIa is a serine protease that complexes with TF to proteolytically cleave and activate factor X. In turn, factor X complexes with factor Va to cleave prothrombin, yielding prothrombin fragment 1+2 (F1+2) and thrombin. As well as activating factor X, the factor VIIa/TF complex also cleaves factor IX (see **Figure 1**). This reaction leads to further thrombin generation as factors IXa and VIIIa together activate more factor X. This is an important reinforcement reaction that is essential for normal hemostasis, as deficiency of either factor VIII (hemophilia A) or factor IX (hemophilia B) lead to severe bleeding diathesis.

Further consolidation reactions take place, including the activation of factors V, VIII, and XI by thrombin. Factors Va and VIIIa act as cofactors for factors Xa and IXa, respectively. Activated factor XI generates more factor IXa.

Another protein that plays an important role in support of coagulation is von Willebrand factor (vWF). This glycoprotein circulates in the form of large multimers, serves a carrier function for factor VIII, and is involved in platelet aggregation [13].

Many of the serine proteinases – factors VII, IX, X, and prothrombin – undergo vitamin K-dependent posttranslational carboxylation of glutamic acid residues to produce γ-carboxyglutamic acid (Gla) [14]. Calcium mediates binding of Gla residues to negatively charged phospholipids – such as phosphatidylserine – exposed on the platelet membrane on activation. Localization of these vitamin K-dependent factors to the platelet membrane greatly enhances the catalytic efficiency of proteolytic reactions.

Inhibition of coagulation

No enzymatic system with such explosive catalytic activity as the coagulation cascade could exist without naturally occurring inhibitors to keep enzymatic activity under control. Inhibitors of the coagulation cascade include:

- TFPI – a direct competitive inhibitor of factors Xa, VIIa, and TF

- antithrombin – irreversibly binds to thrombin, and factors Xa, IXa, and XIa

- activated protein C – inactivates factors Va and VIIIa by proteolytic cleavage in the presence of protein S

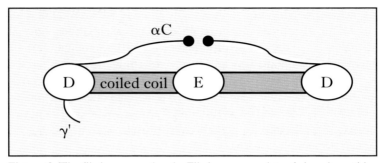

Figure 3. The fibrinogen molecule. Fibrinogen consists of six polypeptides ($A\alpha_2B\beta_2\gamma_2$), which are arranged into a protein with bilateral symmetry. The amino termini of all six chains are located in the central E region, the carboxy termini of the $B\beta$– and γ-chains are located in the D regions, and the carboxy terminus of the $A\alpha$-chain forms a protrusion from the molecule ending in a globular domain (αC). Fibrinopeptides A and B are found in the E region. Cleavage of these peptides exposes binding sites for complementary binding pockets in the D region. The γ-chain is subject to alternative mRNA splicing, resulting in an elongation of the γ-chain (γ') that contains thrombin and factor XIII binding sites.

Formation of crosslinked fibrin

Fibrinogen is a large glycoprotein composed of six polypeptide chains ($A\alpha_2B\beta_2\gamma_2$) arranged into a molecule with bilateral symmetry (see **Figure 3**) [15]. Conversion of fibrinogen into fibrin involves cleavage of fibrinopeptides A and B (FPA and FPB) from the N-terminus of the $A\alpha$- and $B\beta$-chains of fibrinogen, respectively. Cleavage of the fibrinopeptides exposes a binding site on the central E-region of the molecule, which interacts with binding pockets on the distal or D-regions. This interaction leads to the formation of half-staggered, overlapping protofibrils (see **Figure 4**).

FPA is released from fibrinogen at a faster rate than FPB; protofibril formation starts as soon as FPA is released. FPB release is associated with lateral aggregation of the protofibrils into thicker fiber bundles [16,17]. The fibers branch out, forming a 3-dimensional network to which platelets and other proteins – such

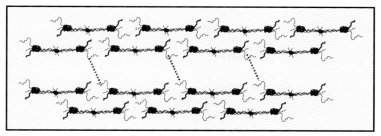

Figure 4. Fibrin polymerization. Binding between sites on the D and E regions exposed by thrombin cleavage of the fibrinopeptides leads to protofibrils of overlapping, half-staggered fibrin monomers. Protofibrils aggregate laterally to form thicker fibers through interaction of the αC-domains, as indicated by dark broken lines.

as albumin and fibronectin – adhere. This forms the structural basis of the blood clot.

Fibrin is covalently crosslinked by factor XIIIa – a protransglutaminase that, when activated by thrombin, catalyses the formation of covalent γ-glutamyl-ε-lysine bonds [18]. Crosslinking occurs between the γ- and α-chains of the fibrin molecule, and greatly enhances the chemical and physical stability of the clot. In addition, factor XIIIa crosslinks α_2-antiplasmin to the α-chain of fibrin, increasing the resistance of the clot to fibrinolysis [19].

Crosslinking by factor XIIIa is closely regulated by formation of the fibrin clot itself, as polymerizing fibrin is a potent enhancer of factor XIII activation by thrombin – an effect that is lost once fibrin is crosslinked [20,21].

Fibrinolysis

A natural defense system against deposition of crosslinked fibrin exists *in vivo* to maintain vascular patency. This system involves proteolytic breakdown of (crosslinked) fibrin, and, like the coagulation cascade, it is based on a series of serine proteinase reactions (see **Figure 5**). Plasmin is central to the process of

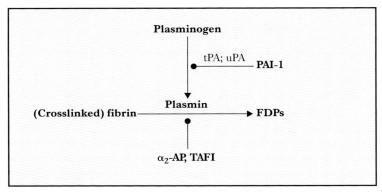

Figure 5. The fibrinolysis pathway. Crosslinked fibrin is broken down by plasmin generated by endogenous or pharmacological plasminogen activation. α_2-AP: α_2-antiplasmin; FDP: fibrin degradation product; PAI-1: plasminogen activator inhibitor-1; TAFI: thrombin-activatable fibrinolysis inhibitor; tPA: tissue-type plasminogen activator; uPA: urokinase-type plasminogen activator.

fibrinolysis. This serine proteinase degrades fibrin by cleaving a number of peptide bonds in the αC-connecting peptide and the coiled-coil region of the protein, forming fragment E- and D-dimers and other degradation products [22].

Plasminogen is converted into plasmin by cleavage of the Arg_{561}–Val_{562} peptide bond by two structurally similar but immunologically distinct plasminogen activators – tissue-type plasminogen activator (tPA) and urokinase-type plasminogen activator (uPA) [23]. Both tPA and uPA also belong to the serine proteinase family. Fibrin C-terminal lysine residues regulate the activation of plasminogen by tPA; tPA has poor enzyme activity in the absence of fibrin. The uPA-mediated activation of plasminogen is regulated by the binding of uPA to a cellular receptor (uPAR) that functions as a cofactor for the conversion [24].

In addition to the above interactions, the fibrinolytic system is regulated further by three inhibitors (see **Figure 5**):

- α_2-antiplasmin – the main physiological inhibitor of plasmin that binds to the active site and forms a 1:1 stoichiometric complex with the enzyme [25]

- plasminogen activator inhibitor (PAI)-1 – a glycoprotein of the serpin family that inhibits tPA and uPA [26]

- thrombin-activatable fibrinolysis inhibitor (TAFI) – a newly discovered carboxypeptidase that reduces the affinity of plasminogen for its substrate, fibrin, by cleaving the C-terminal lysines to which plasminogen binds [27]. In addition, activated TAFI inhibits plasmin generation catalyzed by a complex of tPA and fibrin degradation product E [28]

Cellular interactions

Blood cells provide many of the proteins involved in hemostasis, as well as the surface where crucial enzyme and ligand–receptor reactions occur. Thrombosis in the venous system occurs under low-flow conditions, and results in the formation of an erythrocyte-rich fibrin clot. Thrombi in the arterial vascular bed are platelet-rich and are formed under conditions of high-shear stress.

Platelets

Blood platelets are small, discoid, anucleoid cells that adhere to collagen – exposed after vessel injury – to form a primary hemostatic plug. They are further activated when thrombin, generated by the coagulation cascade, proteolytically cleaves two members of the proteinase-activated receptor (PAR) family exposed on the platelet surface: PAR-1 and PAR-4 [29]. Upon activation, platelets lose their typical discoid shape and become irregular in appearance, form pseudopods, and release the contents of α-granules. These granules contain a rich mixture of prothrombotic factors – including calcium, fibrinogen, factor V, vWF, factor XI, kininogen, and PAI-1 – as well as adhesive proteins – such as thrombospondin, fibronectin, and vitronectin [30]. Platelet adhesion occurs via an interaction between collagen, vWF, and the platelet receptor glycoprotein (GP)Ib-IX.

Fibrin is generated around the platelet aggregates and interacts with GPIIb/IIIa receptors [31].

The platelet membrane undergoes a change during activation whereby negatively charged phospholipids – such as phosphatidylserine – that are normally situated on the cytoplasmic side of the membrane move to the extracellular side [32]. This cellular reaction is also referred to as membrane flip-flop, and it provides the surface to which vitamin K-dependent coagulation factors bind in the presence of calcium, increasing the catalytic efficiency of proteolysis.

Membrane flip-flop, α-granule release, and aggregation/adhesion make platelets a critical element in blood clotting, and their role in thrombosis is illustrated by the efficacy of GPIIb/IIIa inhibition in the management of cardiovascular disease (CVD).

Endothelium

Under normal conditions, the vascular endothelium maintains anticoagulant properties to prevent intravascular clotting. There are two major anticoagulant mechanisms at work on the endothelium.

The first mechanism involves the proteoglycan layer that covers the luminal surface of the endothelium. Proteoglycans bind and enhance the anticoagulant activity of TFPI and antithrombin. The majority of the TFPI vascular pool (>75%) is bound to the endothelial proteoglycans, localizing it to the vascular lining. This endothelial-bound TFPI can be released by injection of heparin [33].

The second major anticoagulant mechanism is maintained by the expression of thrombomodulin – an endothelial transmembrane protein that binds thrombin and alters its specificity from procoagulant to anticoagulant. The thrombin–thrombomodulin complex is also the main activator of protein C [34]. Lesions on the endothelium expose the procoagulant subendothelium, which is rich in TF. In addition, perturbations under inflammatory conditions induce the expression of TF by endothelial cells and monocytes. Therefore, under certain pathological conditions, the endothelium can display a thrombogenic phenotype.

Current developments in our understanding of hemostasis

A number of novel cellular receptors for coagulation factors have been identified – such as endothelial protein C receptor (EPCR), which functions as a receptor and cofactor of activated protein C [35], and the PAR family of receptors, which play a role in thrombin-dependent platelet activation [29]. The receptor activity of TF has also been investigated [36].

A novel metalloproteinase belonging to the ADAMTS family – ADAMTS13 – is responsible for cleaving vWF to produce a typical large multimer pattern [37]. Deficiency of ADAMTS13 leads to an abnormal number of high-molecular weight multimers, and is associated with a greater risk of developing thrombotic thrombocytopenia [37,38].

The genetics of hemostasis and related disorders of thrombosis has been a major topic of study in the last decade, and this has led to the discovery of interesting single nucleotide polymorphisms (SNPs). An example is the factor V Leiden mutation, which is an SNP in the protein C cleavage site of factor V. This mutation makes factor V resistant to inactivation by protein C, and increases the risk of developing deep vein thrombosis [39]. Numerous other SNPs in genes involved in hemostasis have been described; however, most show inconsistent associations with the clinical manifestations of thrombosis.

Metabolic determinants of thrombotic risk in diabetes

Diabetes mellitus is characterized by hyperglycemia and the chronic development of vascular complications. Although the underlying pathogenesis of type 1 and type 2 diabetes differs, both are associated with micro- and macrovascular disorders. Improvements in glycemic control ameliorate the development and progression of microvascular complications, and there is evidence that macrovascular disease is also reduced by tighter glycemic control, although probably to a lesser extent. There are many candidates for the mechanisms that translate poor glycemic control into vascular disorders – including changes in hemostasis, protein glycosylation, the formation of advanced glycation endproducts (AGEs), oxidative stress, inflammation, and lipid abnormalities.

Hemostasis

A variety of hemostatic abnormalities are associated with diabetes, including increases in vWF, factors VII, VIII, and X, and fibrinogen [40–43], and prothrombotic alterations in the coagulation inhibitors protein C and antithrombin [44]. Profound suppression of the fibrinolytic pathway, reflected by elevated PAI-1 concentrations, occurs in type 2 diabetes mellitus (T2DM) patients in association with underlying insulin resistance [45].

Insulin and insulin resistance

Metabolic disturbances associated with insulin resistance are common in the general population, with an estimated prevalence of around 25% (see **Figure 6**) [46]. A spectrum of related metabolic disorders are recognized, including T2DM, impaired glucose tolerance, and compensated normal glucose tolerance. The metabolic features of insulin resistance are associated with hyperglycemia, hypertension, hypertriglyceridemia, a decrease in high-density lipoprotein cholesterol, and an increase in low-density lipoproteins (see **Table 1**). There is evidence that fibrinogen, PAI-1, factor VII, and vWF are associated to a varying degree with features of the insulin resistance syndrome and therefore increase with the metabolic features (see **Table 1**) [47,48]. Both glycosylated hemoglobin and body-mass index have been related to increased fibrinogen concentrations [49].

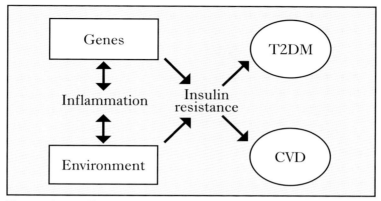

Figure 6. Insulin resistance and thrombotic risk. Insulin resistance associates with inflammatory, hemostatic, and vascular changes that increase the risk for cardiovascular disease (CVD). The metabolic syndrome associated with insulin resistance is influenced by genetic and environmental factors that may be modulated by inflammation. T2DM: type 2 diabetes mellitus.

Fibrinolysis is markedly different in subjects with type 1 and type 2 diabetes (see **Table 2**). Patients with T2DM experience a profound suppression of fibrinolysis due to increased levels of PAI-1 [45]. Several studies have noted the strong relationship between features of the T2DM metabolic syndrome and elevated PAI-1 levels (see **Table 1**). In particular, PAI-1 correlates with triglyceride concentrations [45,50]. The promoter of the PAI-1 gene contains a triglyceride-responsive element; PAI-1 gene expression is elevated with high levels of triglycerides. In patients with type 1 diabetes (T1DM), there is no consistent defect in fibrinolysis. Studies suggest that T1DM patients have an increase in basal fibrinolytic activity and tPA concentrations, with normal or reduced levels of PAI-1 [51,52].

Several studies have reported increased factor VII in T2DM patients with microalbuminuria or without evidence of complications [53,54]. In T1DM patients, factor VII is elevated with microalbuminuria, although a study in twins with T1DM found reduced levels of factor VII [55,56]. The major determinants of

Metabolic features	Prothrombotic/antifibrinolytic features
Hyperglycemia	↑ PAI-1
Hyperinsulinemia	↑ Fibrinogen
Hypertension	↑ Factor VII
Hypertriglyceridemia	↑ von Willebrand factor
Hyperuricemia	
↓ HDL-cholesterol	

Table 1. Characteristics of insulin resistance. HDL: high-density lipoprotein; LDL: low-density lipoprotein; PAI-1: plasminogen activator inhibitor-1; ↑: increased expression; ↓: decreased expression.

factor VII concentration appear to be gender, microalbuminuria, and some features of the insulin resistance syndrome. In nondiabetic populations, there is evidence that factor VII is related to cholesterol and triglyceride concentrations [57]. These findings indicate that elevated factor VII clusters with insulin resistance in a manner similar to that described for PAI-1 (see **Table 2**).

Glucose and advanced glycation endproducts

DCCT (the Diabetes Control and Complications Trial) demonstrated that improvements in glycemic control and protein glycation ameliorate the development and progression of microvascular complications [58]. Evidence indicates that minor increases in blood glucose, previously thought to be harmless, are associated with subtle alterations in cardiac function and result in increases in mortality from ischemic heart disease [59]. Prolonged exposure of proteins to high glucose concentrations leads to nonenzymatic glycation, and ultimately to the irreversible production of AGEs. A number of scavenger receptors for AGEs exist, including RAGE (receptor for advanced glycation endproducts). Binding of AGEs to RAGE sets off a cascade of

	Type 1 diabetes	Type 2 diabetes
Fibrinogen	↑ or ↓	↑
Factor VII	↑ or ↓	↑
von Willebrand factor	↑	↑
Antithrombin	↓	↓
Protein C	→ or ↓	→ or ↓
PAI-1	→ or ↑ or ↓	↑

Table 2. Changes of hemostasis in type 1 and type 2 diabetes. PAI-1: plasminogen activator inhibitor-1; ↑: increased; ↓: decreased; →: no change.

intracellular messages that lead to oxidative stress, increased expression of adhesion molecules – such as vascular cell adhesion molecule (VCAM)-1 – and hemostatic proteins – such as TF, vWF, and PAI-1 [60]. Evidence from animal models indicates that soluble RAGE prevents the development of atheroma [61].

Patients with both type 1 and type 2 diabetes experience glycation of fibrinogen, and the degree of glycation correlates with glycemic control. Enzymatic glycosylation of fibrinogen – mediated by glycosyl transferase – takes place in the Golgi apparatus prior to the secretion of fibrinogen and plays a role in determining the structure and function of the fibrin clot [62]. It is also possible that nonenzymatic glycation influences fibrin structure and function, because *in vitro* glycation of fibrinogen alters the binding affinity of tPA and plasminogen for fibrin and reduces fibrinolysis [63,64].

Risk of thrombosis and vascular disease in diabetes

Vascular complications of diabetes affect the microvasculature (eyes, nerves, and kidney) and macrovasculature (the cardiovascular system) trees. Some of the underlying mechanisms involved in both micro- and macrovascular complications appear to be related to the development of insulin resistance, which is associated with a clustering of atheromatous risk factors (see **Table 1**). The development of microalbuminuria is associated with a progression of insulin resistance and an increase in the severity of atherothrombotic risk. As insulin resistance progresses to frank diabetes, there are increases in the formation of AGEs, the interactions between AGEs and RAGE, and prothrombotic interactions; consequently, the risk of both macro- and microvascular complications is increased.

Microvascular disease

Development of microvascular complications involves increased vascular permeability and blood flow, basement membrane thickening, capillary occlusion, microaneurysm formation, and angiogenesis. There is evidence that the fibrinolytic system, which regulates plasmin generation and local thrombus formation, has an important role in neovascularization [65,66]. Ischemic changes and associated hypoxia lead to increased expression of genes in the retinal vasculature – including vascular endothelial growth factor (VEGF) [67]. VEGF may play a role in the stimulation of prothrombotic elements in the blood.

Nephropathy

Type 1 and type 2 diabetics with microalbuminuria have increases in plasma fibrinogen [68,69], fibrin monomers [70], and urinary fibrinogen degradation products [71]. Additionally, T1DM patients with microalbuminuria have elevated F1+2 levels; this correlates with the transcapillary escape rate [72]. There is also evidence that platelet activation and vWF are involved in nephropathy [73,74]. Patients with microalbuminuria have elevated vWF levels, and there are indications that high vWF levels precede the development of microalbuminuria by 3 years [75,76].

Retinopathy

It is difficult to disentangle nephropathy and retinopathy in diabetic subjects, as it is invariable that subjects with established nephropathy will have some form of retinopathy. As well as being related to the deterioration of renal function, hyperinsulinemia has been linked to retinopathy through insulin effects on endothelial cell proliferation [77]. This is presumably due to the release of VEGF, as VEGF antibodies block the effect [65,67,77]. AGEs release PAI-1 and TF from endothelial cells, and it has been hypothesized that both angiogenesis (mediated by VEGF) and thrombosis with focal ischemia (mediated by PAI-1) may contribute to the development of retinopathy [65,67,77]. Increased levels of TF have been described in T2DM subjects with retinopathy, and there is evidence that this patient subcategory experiences activation of coagulation with increased FPA plasma levels [78,79].

Neuropathy

Studies have indicated that increased platelet activation occurs with elevated levels of vWF [74,80–82]. In a prospective study of 63 young diabetic subjects, baseline vWF antigen and activity were significantly higher in eight patients with evidence of neuropathy [83]. This suggests that endothelial dysfunction – demonstrated by high vWF levels – may be associated with the development of neuropathy in young patients.

Macrovascular disease

Macrovascular complications – coronary artery disease (CAD), cerebrovascular disease, and peripheral vascular disease – lead to the majority of the early mortality associated with diabetes; approximately 70% of T2DM patients will die from CAD. Fibrinogen levels are elevated in T2DM patients compared with controls [44,56,84]. Prospective studies in nondiabetic cohorts have demonstrated a strong relationship between high levels of fibrinogen and the development of CAD and cerebrovascular disease [85]. In the Northwick Park Heart Study, fibrinogen was more strongly associated with CAD than cholesterol [86]. There have been no prospective studies of fibrinogen in relation to vascular disorders in diabetic subjects, but it is likely that hyperfibrinogenemia plays a similar role in these patients.

The Northwick Park Heart Study reported that global suppression of fibrinolysis was related to subsequent risk for myocardial infarction (MI) [86]. Hamsten et al. found that levels of PAI-1 activity 3 months after a first MI in young men could be used to predict recurrent MI [87]. The Physicians' Health Study proposed that tPA was independently associated with stroke in a large study of American physicians [88]. Although more controversial, there is also evidence that other proteins related to insulin resistance – including factors VII and XII – play a role in the risk for CAD and MI [86,89–91].

Therapeutic implications of thrombotic risk

Thrombotic and fibrinolytic processes play a pivotal role in the development of vascular disease; this statement is reinforced by the observation that many drugs that are active in these systems radically alter outcome. Some of these drugs are direct acting, such as antiplatelet agents – aspirin, clopidogrel, and GPIIb/IIIa inhibitors – or fibrinolytic agents – such as streptokinase and tPA. Therapies that reduce insulin resistance in T2DM – such as metformin and thiazolidinediones – also have indirect beneficial effects on the prothrombotic profile due to the strong association between insulin resistance and thrombotic risk clustering [92].

Therapy for the thrombotic complications associated with diabetes will take several different directions in the future. Intensive research has allowed a deeper understanding of the processes involved in thrombosis. The development of RNA aptamers and specific inhibitors of thrombotic processes will represent major advances for the management of macrovascular disease [93]. The awareness that cardiovascular disease and T2DM are the same condition, with evidence of pleiotropy between vascular risk and insulin resistance, raises the possibility that other insulin-resistance lowering agents will indirectly ameliorate vascular risk and the risk for T2DM. Many tools have been developed – such as computational chemistry, bioinformatics, pharmacogenomics, and gene transfer – that will support the development of novel therapeutics in this field. The

Doomsday scenario of 300 million diabetic subjects worldwide by the year 2025 – with 70% dying from cardiovascular complications – necessitates the use of the new opportunities that are available to prevent diabetes and its complications.

Conclusion

Diabetes mellitus is associated with a huge burden of micro- and macrovascular complications. Evidence exists to implicate abnormalities in hemostasis in the pathogenesis of all vascular phenotypes associated with diabetes; this association is strongest for CAD and T2DM. Around 200 million individuals worldwide currently carry a diagnosis of diabetes; the vast majority (more than 98%) of these individuals have T2DM. The cause of the tight association between diabetes and CAD is uncertain, but it has been suggested that common genetic and environmental antecedents underpin both conditions (the Common Soil Hypothesis) [94]. Recent studies have indicated that proinflammatory responses, which are candidates for the common causation of both insulin resistance and vascular disease, are associated with diabetes and CAD [95,96]. Toxic environmental influences – such as smoking, oxidized low-density lipoproteins, hyperglycemia, AGE/RAGE interactions, and physical inactivity – induce proinflammatory responses, insulin resistance, and the associated clustering of vascular risk. Evidence indicates that inflammatory cytokines, complement proteins, and C-reactive protein can have adverse effects on coagulation/fibrinolysis pathways, and endothelial cell and adipocyte function, and may enhance vascular damage and risk for CAD. In both type 1 and type 2 diabetes, an evidence base has been acquired to help prevent the complications associated with poor metabolic control. Understanding the crucial role of prothrombotic pathways will help in the design of better management strategies to prevent the crippling vascular complications of diabetes mellitus.

References

1. Davie EW, Ratnoff OD. Waterfall sequence for intrinsic blood clotting. *Science* 1964;145:1310–2.

2. Macfarlane RG. An enzyme cascade in the blood clotting mechanism, and its function as a biochemical amplifier. *Nature* 1964;202:498–9.

3. Nemerson Y. The reaction between bovine brain tissue factor and factors VII and X. *Biochemistry* 1966;5:601–8.

4. Broze GJ Jr. Tissue factor pathway inhibitor and the revised theory of coagulation. *Ann Rev Med* 1995;46:103–12.

5. Fuhrer G, Gallimore MJ, Heller W et al. Aprotinin in cardiopulmonary bypass – effects on the Hageman factor (FXII) – Kallikrein system and blood loss. *Blood Coagul Fibrinolysis* 1992;3:99–104.

6. Frank RD, Weber J, Dresbach H et al. Role of contact system activation in hemodialyzer-induced thrombogenicity. *Kidney Int* 2001;60:1972–81.

7. Colman RW. Biologic activities of the contact factors *in vivo* – potentiation of hypotension, inflammation, and fibrinolysis, and inhibition of cell adhesion, angiogenesis and thrombosis. *Thromb Haemost* 1999;82:1568–77.

8. Mackman N. Regulation of the tissue factor gene. *Thromb Haemost* 1997;78:747–54.

9. Marmur JD, Thiruvikraman SV, Fyfe BS et al. Identification of active tissue factor in human coronary atheroma. *Circulation* 1996;94:1226–32.

10. Broze GJ Jr, Warren LA, Novotny WF et al. The lipoprotein-associated coagulation inhibitor that inhibits the factor VII-tissue factor complex also inhibits factor Xa: insight into its possible mechanism of action. *Blood* 1988;71:335–43.

11. Giesen PL, Rauch U, Bohrmann B et al. Blood-borne tissue factor: another view of thrombosis. *Proc Natl Acad Sci USA* 1999;96:2311–5.

12. Balasubramanian V, Grabowski E, Bini A et al. Platelets, circulating tissue factor, and fibrin colocalize in *ex vivo* thrombi: real-time fluorescence images of thrombus formation and propagation under defined flow conditions. *Blood* 2002;100:2787–92.

13. Ruggeri ZM. Structure and function of von Willebrand factor. *Thromb Haemost* 1999;82:576–84.

14. Vermeer C. Gamma-carboxyglutamate-containing proteins and the vitamin K-dependent carboxylase. *Biochem J* 1990;266:625–36.

15. Matsuda M. Structure and function of fibrinogen inferred from hereditary dysfibrinogens. *Int J Hematol* 2000;72:436–47.

16. Mullin JL, Gorkun OV, Lord ST. Decreased lateral aggregation of a variant recombinant fibrinogen provides insight into the polymerisation mechanism. *Biochemistry* 2000;39:9843–9.

17. Weisel JW, Veklich Y, Gorkun OV. The sequence of cleavage of fibrinopeptides from fibrinogen is important for protofibril formation and enhancement of lateral aggregation in fibrin clots. *J Mol Biol* 1993;232:285–97.

18. Lorand L. Sol Sherry Lecture in Thrombosis: research on clot stabilization provides clues for improving thrombolytic therapies. *Arterioscler Thromb Vasc Biol* 2000;20:2–9.

19. Sakata Y, Aoki N. Cross-linking of alpha 2-plasmin inhibitor to fibrin by fibrin-stabilizing factor. *J Clin Invest* 1980;65:290–7.

20. Greenberg CS, Miraglia CC. The effect of fibrin polymers on thrombin-catalyzed plasma factor XIIIa formation. *Blood* 1985;66:466–9.

21. Hornyak TJ, Shafer JA. Interactions of factor XIII with fibrin as substrate and cofactor. *Biochemistry* 1992;31:423–9.

22. Gaffney PJ. Fibrin degradation products. A review of structures found *in vitro* and *in vivo*. *Ann NY Acad Sci* 2001;936:594–610.

23. Stump DC, Lijnen HR, Collen D. Purification and characterization of a novel low molecular weight form of single-chain urokinase-type plasminogen activator. *J Biol Chem* 1986;261:17120–6.

24. Ellis V, Behrendt N, Dano K. Plasminogen activation by receptor-bound urokinase. A kinetic study with both cell-associated and isolated receptor. *J Biol Chem* 1991;266:12752–8.

25. Wiman B, Collen D. On the mechanism of the reaction between human alpha$_2$ - antiplasmin and plasmin. *J Biol Chem* 1979;254:9291–7.

26. Kruithof EK, Tran-Thang C, Ransijn A et al. Demonstration of a fast-acting inhibitor of plasminogen activators in human plasma. *Blood* 1984;64:907–13.

27. Bajzar L, Manuel R, Nesheim ME. Purification and characterization of TAFI, a thrombin-activable fibrinolysis inhibitor. *J Biol Chem* 1995;270:14477–84.

28. Stewart RJ, Fredenburgh JC, Rischke JA et al. Thrombin-activable fibrinolysis inhibitor attenuates (DD)E-mediated stimulation of plasminogen activation by reducing the affinity of (DD)E for tissue plasminogen activator. A potential mechanism for enhancing the fibrin specificity of tissue plasminogen activator. *J Biol Chem* 2000;275:36612–20.

29. Macfarlane SR, Seatter MJ, Kanke T et al. Proteinase-activated receptors. *Pharmacol Rev* 2001;53:245–82.

30. Rendu F, Brohard-Bohn B. The platelet release reaction: granules' constituents, secretion and functions. *Platelets* 2001;12:261–73.

31. Phillips DR, Charo IF, Scarborough RM. GPIIb-IIIa: the responsive integrin. *Cell* 1991;65:359–62.

32. Comfurius P, Williamson P, Smeets EF et al. Reconstitution of phospholipid scramblase activity from human blood platelets. *Biochemistry* 1996;35:7631–4.

33. Holst J, Lindblad B, Bergqvist D et al. The effect of protamine sulphate on plasma tissue factor pathway inhibitor released by intravenous and subcutaneous unfractionated and low molecular weight heparin in man. *Thromb Res* 1997;86:343–8.

34. Esmon CT, Owen WG. Identification of an endothelial cell cofactor for thrombin-catalyzed activation of protein C. *Proc Natl Acad Sci USA* 1981;78:2249–52.

35. Oganesyan V, Oganesyan N, Terzyan S et al. The crystal structure of the endothelial protein C receptor and a bound phospholipid. *J Biol Chem* 2002;277:24851–4.

36. Morrissey JH. Tissue factor: an enzyme cofactor and a true receptor. *Thromb Haemost* 2001;86:66–74.

37. Levy GG, Nichols WC, Lian EC et al. Mutations in a member of the ADAMTS gene family cause thrombotic thrombocytopenic purpura. *Nature* 2001;413:488–94.

38. Kokame K, Matsumoto M, Soejima K et al. Mutations and common polymorphisms in ADAMTS13 gene responsible for von Willebrand factor-cleaving protease activity. *Proc Natl Acad Sci USA* 2002;99:11902–7.

39. Bertina RM, Koeleman BP, Koster T et al. Mutation in blood coagulation factor V associated with resistance to activated protein C. *Nature* 1994;369:64–7.

40. Conlan MG, Folsom AR, Finch A et al. Associations of factor VIII and von Willebrand factor with age, race, sex, and risk factors for atherosclerosis. The Atherosclerosis Risk in Communities (ARIC) Study. *Thromb Haemost* 1993;70:380–5.

41. Fuller JH, Keen H, Jarrett RJ et al. Haemostatic variables associated with diabetes and its complications. *BMJ* 1979;2:964–6.

42. el Khawand C, Jamart J, Donckier J et al. Hemostasis variables in type I diabetic patients without demonstrable vascular complications. *Diabetes Care* 1993;16:1137–45.

43. Juhan-Vague I, Alessi MC, Vague P. Thrombogenic and fibrinolytic factors and cardiovascular risk in non- insulin-dependent diabetes mellitus. *Ann Med* 1996;28:371–80.

44. Kwaan HC. Changes in blood coagulation, platelet function, and plasminogen- plasmin system in diabetes. *Diabetes* 1992;41 (Suppl. 2):32–5.

45. Juhan-Vague I, Alessi MC, Vague P. Increased plasma plasminogen activator inhibitor 1
     levels. A possible link between insulin resistance and atherothrombosis. *Diabetologia*
     1991;34:457–62.
46. Eriksson J, Taimela S, Koivisto VA. Exercise and the metabolic syndrome. *Diabetologia*
     1997;40:125–35.
47. Burchfiel CM, Curb JD, Sharp DS et al. Distribution and correlates of insulin in elderly
     men. The Honolulu Heart Program. *Arterioscler Thromb Vasc Biol* 1995;15:2213–21.
48. Mansfield MW, Heywood DM, Grant PJ. Circulating levels of factor VII, fibrinogen, and
     von Willebrand factor and features of insulin resistance in first-degree relatives of
     patients with NIDDM. *Circulation* 1996;94:2171–6.
49. Vanninen E, Laitinen J, Uusitupa M. Physical activity and fibrinogen concentration in
     newly diagnosed NIDDM. *Diabetes Care* 1994;17:1031–8.
50. Grant PJ. Polymorphisms of coagulation/fibrinolysis genes: gene environment
     interactions and vascular risk. *Prostaglandins Leukot Essent Fatty Acids* 1997;57:473–7.
51. Gough SC, Grant PJ. The fibrinolytic system in diabetes mellitus. *Diabet Med*
     1991;8:898–905.
52. Walmsley D, Hampton KK, Grant PJ. Contrasting fibrinolytic responses in type 1
     (insulin-dependent) and type 2 (non-insulin-dependent) diabetes. *Diabet Med*
     1991;8:954–9.
53. Kario K, Matsuo T, Kobayashi H et al. Activation of tissue factor-induced coagulation
     and endothelial cell dysfunction in non-insulin-dependent diabetic patients with
     microalbuminuria. *Arterioscler Thromb Vasc Biol* 1995;15:1114–20.
54. Knobl P, Schernthaner G, Schnack C et al. Haemostatic abnormalities persist despite
     glycaemic improvement by insulin therapy in lean type 2 diabetic patients. *Thromb
     Haemost* 1994;71:692–7.
55. Gruden G, Cavallo-Perin P, Bazzan M et al. PAI-1 and factor VII activity are higher in
     IDDM patients with microalbuminuria. *Diabetes* 1994;43:426–9.
56. Dubrey SW, Reaveley DR, Seed M et al. Risk factors for cardiovascular disease in IDDM.
     A study of identical twins. *Diabetes* 1994;43:831–5.
57. Miller GJ, Martin JC, Mitropoulos KA et al. Plasma factor VII is activated by postprandial
     triglyceridaemia, irrespective of dietary fat composition. *Atherosclerosis* 1991;86:163–71.
58. DCCT writing team. Effect of intensive therapy on the microvascular complications
     of type 1 diabetes mellitus. *JAMA* 2002;287:2563–9.
59. Donahue RP, Abbott RD, Reed DM et al. Postchallenge glucose concentration and
     coronary heart disease in men of Japanese ancestry. Honolulu Heart Program. *Diabetes*
     1987;36:689–92.
60. Yamagishi S, Fujimori H, Yonekura H et al. Advanced glycation endproducts inhibit
     prostacyclin production and induce plasminogen activator inhibitor-1 in human
     microvascular endothelial cells. *Diabetologia* 1998;41:1435–41.
61. Park L, Raman KG, Lee KJ et al. Suppression of accelerated diabetic atherosclerosis
     by the soluble receptor for advanced glycation endproducts. *Nat Med* 1998;4:1025–31.
62. Langer BG, Weisel JW, Dinauer PA et al. Deglycosylation of fibrinogen accelerates
     polymerization and increases lateral aggregation of fibrin fibers. *J Biol Chem*
     1988;263:15056–63.
63. Bobbink IW, Tekelenburg WL, Sixma JJ et al. Glycated proteins modulate tissue-
     plasminogen activator-catalyzed plasminogen activation. *Biochem Biophys Res Commun*
     1997;240:595–601.
64. Brownlee M, Vlassara H, Cerami A. Nonenzymatic glycosylation reduces the
     susceptibility of fibrin to degradation by plasmin. *Diabetes* 1983;32:680–4.
65. Lansink M, Koolwijk P, van Hinsbergh V et al. Effect of steroid hormones and retinoids
     on the formation of capillary-like tubular structures of human microvascular endothelial
     cells in fibrin matrices is related to urokinase expression. *Blood* 1998;92:927–38.

66. Carmeliet P, Moons L, Dewerchin M et al. Insights in vessel development and vascular disorders using targeted inactivation and transfer of vascular endothelial growth factor, the tissue factor receptor, and the plasminogen system. *Ann NY Acad Sci* 1997; 811:191–206.

67. Yamagishi S, Kawakami T, Fujimori H et al. Insulin stimulates the growth and tube formation of human microvascular endothelial cells through autocrine vascular endothelial growth factor. *Microvasc Res* 1999;57:329–39.

68. Bruno G, Cavallo-Perin P, Bargero G et al. Association of fibrinogen with glycemic control and albumin excretion rate in patients with non-insulin-dependent diabetes mellitus. *Ann Intern Med* 1996;125:653–7.

69. Knobl P, Schernthaner G, Schnack C et al. Thrombogenic factors are related to urinary albumin excretion rate in type 1 (insulin-dependent) and type 2 (non-insulin-dependent) diabetic patients. *Diabetologia* 1993;36:1045–50.

70. Sumida Y, Wada H, Fujii M et al. Increased soluble fibrin monomer and soluble thrombomodulin levels in non-insulin-dependent diabetes mellitus. *Blood Coagul Fibrinolysis* 1997;8:303–7.

71. Shibata T, Magari Y, Kamberi P et al. Significance of urinary fibrin/fibrinogen degradation products (FDP) D-dimer measured by a highly sensitive ELISA method with a new monoclonal antibody (D-D E72) in various renal diseases. *Clin Nephrol* 1995;44:91–5.

72. Myrup B, Rossing P, Jensen T et al. Procoagulant activity and intimal dysfunction in IDDM. *Diabetologia* 1995;38:73–8.

73. Iwase E, Tawata M, Aida K et al. A cross-sectional evaluation of spontaneous platelet aggregation in relation to complications in patients with type II diabetes mellitus. *Metabolism* 1998;47:699–705.

74. Omoto S, Nomura S, Shouzu A et al. Significance of platelet-derived microparticles and activated platelets in diabetic nephropathy. *Nephron* 1999;81:271–7.

75. Stehouwer CD, Fischer HR, van Kuijk AW et al. Endothelial dysfunction precedes development of microalbuminuria in IDDM. *Diabetes* 1995;44:561–4.

76. Myrup B, Mathiesen ER, Ronn B et al. Endothelial function and serum lipids in the course of developing microalbuminuria in insulin-dependent diabetes mellitus. *Diabetes Res* 1994;26:33–9.

77. Kubo M, Kiyohara Y, Kato I et al. Effect of hyperinsulinemia on renal function in a general Japanese population: the Hisayama study. *Kidney Int* 1999;55:2450–6.

78. Zumbach M, Hofmann M, Borcea V et al. Tissue factor antigen is elevated in patients with microvascular complications of diabetes mellitus. *Exp Clin Endocrinol Diabetes* 1997;105:206–12.

79. Roy MS, Podgor MJ, Rick ME. Plasma fibrinopeptide A, beta-thromboglobulin, and platelet factor 4 in diabetic retinopathy. *Invest Ophthalmol Vis Sci* 1988;29:856–60.

80. Rauch U, Ziegler D, Piolot R et al. Platelet activation in diabetic cardiovascular autonomic neuropathy. *Diabet Med* 1999;16:848–52.

81. Ford I, Malik RA, Newrick PG et al. Relationships between haemostatic factors and capillary morphology in human diabetic neuropathy. *Thromb Haemost* 1992;68:628–33.

82. Solerte SB, Fioravanti M, Schifino N et al. Hemorheologic and hemostatic changes in long-standing insulin-dependent (type I) diabetic patients with peripheral and autonomic cardiovascular neuropathy. *Acta Diabetol Lat* 1988;25:235–42.

83. Plater ME, Ford I, Dent MT et al. Elevated von Willebrand factor antigen predicts deterioration in diabetic peripheral nerve function. *Diabetologia* 1996;39:336–43.

84. Lee P, Jenkins A, Bourke C et al. Prothrombotic and antithrombotic factors are elevated in patients with type 1 diabetes complicated by microalbuminuria. *Diabet Med* 1993;10:122–8.

85. Ernst E, Resch KL. Fibrinogen as a cardiovascular risk factor: a meta-analysis and review of the literature. *Ann Intern Med* 1993;118:956–63.

86. Meade TW, North WR, Chakrabarti R et al. Haemostatic function and cardiovascular death: early results of a prospective study. *Lancet* 1980;1:1050–4.

87. Hamsten A, de Faire U, Walldius G et al. Plasminogen activator inhibitor in plasma: risk factor for recurrent myocardial infarction. *Lancet* 1987;2:3–9.

88. Ridker PM, Hennekens CH, Stampfer MJ et al. Prospective study of endogenous tissue plasminogen activator and risk of stroke. *Lancet* 1994;343:940–3.

89. Heinrich J, Balleisen L, Schulte H et al. Fibrinogen and factor VII in the prediction of coronary risk. Results from the PROCAM study in healthy men. *Arterioscler Thromb* 1994;14:54–9.

90. Kohler HP, Carter AM, Stickland MH et al. Levels of activated FXII in survivors of myocardial infarction – association with circulating risk factors and extent of coronary artery disease. *Thromb Haemost* 1998;79:14–8.

91. Zito F, Drummond F, Bujac SR et al. Epidemiological and genetic associations of activated factor XII concentration with factor VII activity, fibrinopeptide A concentration, and risk of coronary heart disease in men. *Circulation* 2000;102:2058–62.

92. UK Prospective Diabetes Study Group. Effect of intensive blood-glucose control with metformin on complications in overweight patients with type 2 diabetes (UKPDS 34). *Lancet* 1988;352:854–65.

93. Rusconi CP, Scardino E, Layzer J et al. RNA aptamers as reversible antagonists of coagulation factor IXa. *Nature* 2002;419:90–4.

94. Stern MP. Diabetes and cardiovascular disease. The "common soil" hypothesis. *Diabetes* 1995;44:369–74.

95. Festa A, D'Agostino R Jr, Tracy RP et al. Elevated levels of acute-phase proteins and plasminogen activator inhibitor-1 predict the development of type 2 diabetes: the insulin resistance atherosclerosis study. *Diabetes* 2002;51:1131–7.

96. Pradhan AD, Ridker PM. Do atherosclerosis and type 2 diabetes share a common inflammatory basis? *Eur Heart J* 2002;23:831–4.

Adjunctive pharmacotherapy

David M Safley

Introduction

With an estimated 16 million people with type 2 diabetes mellitus (T2DM) in the US – and an additional 5 million who remain undiagnosed – diabetes places a huge burden upon the healthcare system. Approximately 10% of total healthcare expenses in the US (25% of Medicare dollars) are allocated to the treatment of T2DM or its associated complications. Despite this large utilization of healthcare resources, age-adjusted death rates for T2DM continue to climb. While the death rates for cardiovascular disease (CVD), stroke, and cancer have remained stable or decreased since 1980, the death rate for T2DM in the US has increased by 30% [1].

A NHANES (National Health and Nutrition Examination Survey) I follow-up study revealed a 36.4% decrease in age-adjusted heart disease mortality in nondiabetic men, but only a 13.1% decrease in men with T2DM between the two sampling periods of 1971–1975 and 1982–1984. The same study revealed a 27% decrease in the age-adjusted heart disease mortality in nondiabetic women, but a dramatic 23% increase in women with T2DM. These findings suggest that people with T2DM remain at heightened risk for CVD [2]. Although there have been recent advances in the event-free survival for patients with CVD, patients with T2DM continue to have unacceptable cardiovascular morbidity and mortality. In fact, CVD accounts for approximately 70% of all case fatalities.

Over the past few years, several clinical trials have been conducted to determine the benefits of specific medications in this patient population in an attempt to define a state-of-the-art therapy for the disease.

Global risk

In MRFIT (the Multiple Risk Factor Intervention Trial), men with T2DM were found to have a 3-fold higher absolute risk for cardiovascular death than nondiabetic men (160 vs. 53 cardiovascular deaths per 10,000 person-years, $P < 0.0001$) – even after controlling for age, race, income, cholesterol levels, blood pressure (BP), and smoking [3].

Many studies have demonstrated the importance of T2DM as a risk factor for cardiovascular morbidity and mortality. In one study, T2DM was shown to be a significant risk factor for cardiovascular death or nonfatal myocardial infarction (MI), along with more traditional risk factors such as the male sex and previous MI [4]. The hemoglobin (Hb)A1c level and duration of diabetes were also major predictors of cardiovascular death or cardiovascular events in this study [4]. Patients with T2DM and no history of coronary heart disease (CHD) have the same risk of suffering an MI as nondiabetic patients who have already had an MI (20.2% vs. 18.8% over 7 years) [5].

In the current era of acute coronary syndrome (ACS) management, people with T2DM remain at increased risk for adverse outcomes compared with nondiabetics. When undergoing coronary stent placement, those with T2DM have higher 6-month adverse event rates – death, MI, and target vessel revascularization – than nondiabetic patients, even with the adjunctive use of a glycoprotein (GP)IIb/IIIa inhibitor or a thienopyridine (odds ratio [OR]: 1.27, $P = 0.02$) [6]. Given this increased risk for atherosclerotic disease, the high case-fatality rate, and the risk of death with the first cardiac event in patients with diabetes, the traditional public health concept of primary versus secondary prevention has been called into question [7].

Associated cardiovascular risk factors

Lifestyle and risk factor modification remains a primary goal for preventing or delaying the onset of CVD. Aggressive control of modifiable risk factors – such as hypertension, dyslipidemia, and blood glucose – leads to a substantial decrease in the risk for cardiovascular morbidity and mortality. Unfortunately, one study found that less than 1% of patients with T2DM who were referred for elective cardiac catheterization had adequate control of all modifiable risk factors: 21% had an HbA1c level >7%; 48% had a low-density lipoprotein (LDL) level >100 mg/dL; and only 10% had their BP controlled to <130/85 mm Hg. Only one of the 235 patients in this study (0.4%) had optimal control of all modifiable risk factors, and over 80% had coronary artery disease (CAD) documented at catheterization [8].

Hypertension

Prevalence in T2DM

There is an increased prevalence of hypertension in the T2DM population. In a study of over 1,500 people with T2DM, 51% were shown to have a BP >140/90 mm Hg [9]. This is much higher than the figure in the general population: NHANES III reported a 20.4% prevalence of BP >140/90 mm Hg.

One of the factors associated with hypertension is advancing age; 35% of white men between the ages of 50 and 69 years have an elevated BP, and this figure rises to 50% for those older than 69 years [10]. Individuals with T2DM, over the age of 60 years, with an elevated BP have double the absolute 5-year risk of suffering a major cardiovascular event than a nondiabetic person of the same age with hypertension. In patients treated with a diuretic, 2.6% of those with T2DM had a major cardiovascular event compared with 0.9% of nondiabetic patients. The same increased risk was observed in those randomized to receive placebo (3.3% vs. 1.0%) [11].

Risk

Control of hypertension in the T2DM population is known to decrease the risk of morbidity and mortality. UKPDS (the United Kingdom Prospective Diabetes Study) 36 examined the relationship between systolic BP (SBP) and vascular complications in T2DM patients. Each 10 mm Hg reduction in SBP was associated with significant decreases in the risk for: MI (relative risk [RR]: 11%, $P < 0.0001$); the combined endpoint of microvascular complications (RR: 10%, $P = 0.0007$); T2DM-related death (RR: 15%, $P < 0.0001$); and all T2DM-related complications (RR: 12%, $P < 0.0001$). The lowest risk was observed in those where treatment decreased the SBP to <120 mm Hg [12].

A meta-analysis performed by the INDIANA (Individual Data Analysis of Antihypertensive Drug Interventions) project evaluated the effect of beta-blockers or diuretics versus placebo in the first-line treatment of hypertension in 1,100 people with T2DM and 15,843 nondiabetic patients. There was a significant decrease in the rate of major cardiovascular events (151 vs. 189 per 1,000 patients $P = 0.032$) and cerebrovascular accidents (CVA) (52 vs. 81 per 1,000 patients, $P = 0.011$) in treated T2DM patients after 1 year. The improved outcomes were less remarkable in the T2DM group than in the nondiabetic group; however, BP reduction was significantly less in the T2DM cohort. Neither group was treated to current Joint National Commission (JNC) guidelines (see below) [13].

The most recent JNC update (JNC-VI) recommends a BP goal of <130/85 mm Hg for all patients, regardless of whether or not they have T2DM. A BP of <120/80 mm Hg is considered "optimal" [14]. In a recent position paper, the American Diabetes Association (ADA) supports targeting a lower BP in patients with T2DM. Their current recommendation is to aim for a goal BP of 130/80 mm Hg – taking into account patient safety [15]. The difference between the two recommendations reflects the impact of clinical trials that were completed during the period between publication of these guidelines. JNC-VI guidelines date from 1997, whereas the ADA recommendations were published in 2002.

Supportive data from the HOT (Hypertension Optimal Treatment) trial demonstrated the benefit of lowering BP beyond the levels recommended by JNC-VI [16]. The incidence of cardiovascular complications in three groups randomly assigned to diastolic BP (DBP) targets of ≤90, ≤85, and ≤80 mm Hg, respectively, was examined. There was a 51% decrease in major cardiovascular events – all MI, all stroke, all other cardiovascular deaths – with DBP targeted to ≤80 mm Hg compared with those treated to a target of ≤90 mm Hg. This 10 mm Hg reduction in DBP resulted in a decrease from 24.4 events per 1,000 patient-years to 11.9 events per 1,000 patient-years ($P = 0.005$ for the trend, RR: 2.06, 95% confidence interval [CI]: 1.24–3.44). This difference was not observed in the group targeted to ≤85 mm Hg. Cardiovascular mortality was also decreased from 11.1 events per 1,000 patient-years to 3.7 events per 1,000 patient-years in the group randomized to the lower BP goal ($P = 0.016$, RR: 3.0, 95% CI: 1.28–7.08) [16].

A cost-effectiveness analysis of the JNC-VI treatment goals found that they compare favorably with other treatment strategies and save money overall in patients aged 60 years or older. In a computer-modeled cohort of high-risk 60-year-old patients, lowering BP from 140/90 mm Hg to 130/85 mm Hg would increase life expectancy from 76.5 years to 77.4 years. Lifetime medical costs would decrease from $59,495 with a BP goal of 140/90 mm Hg to $58,045 with a BP goal of 130/85 mm Hg. Therefore, any treatment that costs less than $414 per year (1996 US dollars) would be cost saving in the long term [17].

It may be necessary to use several medications to meet the BP recommendations of the ADA and JNC-VI. UKPDS 38 determined that almost one third of patients with T2DM required three or more antihypertensive medications after 9 years of follow-up to reach a conservative BP goal of <150/85 mm Hg [18]. Meeting this target BP was associated with a significant reduction in the microvascular complications of: retinopathy (12.0 vs. 19.2 events/1,000 patient-years, $P = 0.0092$); diabetes-related endpoints (sudden death, death from hyper- or hypoglycemia, fatal or nonfatal MI, angina, heart failure, stroke, renal failure, amputation [of at least one digit], vitreous hemorrhage, retinal photocoagulation, blindness in one eye, or cataract extraction) (50.9 vs. 67.4 events/1,000 patient-years, $P = 0.0046$); diabetes-related death (13.7 vs. 20.3 events/1,000 patient-years, $P = 0.019$); and stroke (6.5 vs. 11.6 events/1,000 patient-years, $P = 0.013$). There was a nonsignificant reduction in: all-cause mortality (22.4 vs. 27.2 events/1,000 patient-years, $P = 0.17$); MI (18.6 vs. 23.5 events/1,000 patient-years, $P = 0.13$); and peripheral vascular disease (PVD) (1.4 vs. 2.7 events/1,000 patient-years, $P = 0.17$). These data confirm the importance of controlling hypertension in T2DM patients [18].

Therapy goals

As suggested by the ADA guidelines, the BP treatment target should be ≤130/80 mm Hg. Polypharmacy is commonplace; at least one third of patients will require three or more medications. Considering the results from the HOT, UKPDS 36, and UKPDS 38 trials, a BP target goal of 120/80 mm Hg – rather than a less aggressive goal – is likely to prevent long-term complications. This lower target should be considered for patients at high risk for macrovascular complications of T2DM, including CVD, cerebrovascular disease, and PVD. **Table 1** shows the classes of medications recommended for treatment of hypertension in diabetes. The specific medications used to lower BP are discussed below.

Angiotensin-converting enzyme inhibitors

Angiotensin-converting enzyme (ACE) inhibitors and angiotensin receptor blockers (ARBs), discussed in the next section, act on the renin–angiotensin system. This system has become a major target for antihypertensive therapy. Renin is secreted by the juxtaglomerular apparatus of the kidney in response to decreased perfusion or hypotension. Renin then cleaves angiotensinogen (produced by the liver) to form angiotensin I, which is subsequently converted to angiotensin II by ACE. Angiotensin II increases blood pressure by enhancing aldosterone synthesis, resulting in sodium retention and direct vasoconstriction (see **Figure 1**). The first

---

Hypertension

The BP goal is <130/80 mm Hg; consider a goal of 120/80 mm Hg for individuals at very high risk

Hypertension only – ACE inhibitors, ARBs, beta-blockers, or diuretics

Hypertension with microalbuminuria or nephropathy – ACE inhibitors or ARBs, non-DCCBs if ACE inhibitors/ARBs are not tolerated

With or without hypertension, older than 55 years, with other risk factors – ACE inhibitors

Hypertension with MI – beta-blockers and ACE inhibitors

Table 1. Hypertension treatment: the classes of medications recommended and the stepwise method of adding medications as required to attain a target blood pressure. ACE: angiotensin-converting enzyme, ARB: angiotensin receptor blocker, BP: blood pressure, MI: myocardial infarction, non-DCCB: nondihydropyridine calcium channel blocker.

step in this pathway is inhibited by adrenergic blockers. The third and fourth steps are inhibited by ACE inhibitors and ARBs, respectively [19].

Although many classes of medications are now available for the management of hypertension, ACE inhibitors are the first-line agents for treatment in patients with T2DM. ACE inhibitors have been extensively researched, and have been proven to have an incremental benefit over other medications – even those medications that have similar effects on BP.

The renoprotective benefits of ACE inhibitors have been well documented. In 1993, a meta-analysis of over 100 studies of antihypertensive agents revealed that treatment with ACE inhibitors decreased proteinuria; this decrease was independent of changes in BP, treatment duration, type of diabetes, or stage of nephropathy ($P < 0.0001$) [20]. Reductions in proteinuria due to treatment with other antihypertensive agents can be explained by changes in BP, but ACE inhibitors have an additional beneficial

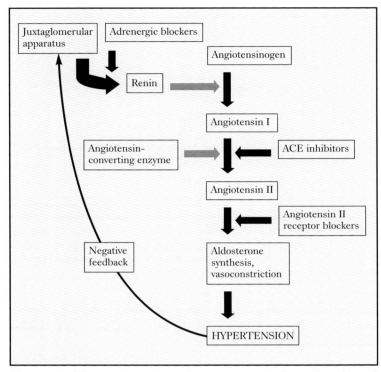

Figure 1. The renin–angiotensin system and sites of action of antihypertensive agents. Black arrows represent the pathway; gray arrows are the sites of enzymatic reactions; orange arrows are the sites of inhibition of the system by pharmacologic agents.

effect on the glomerular filtration rate, independent of BP changes [20].

The beneficial effects of ACE inhibitors have since been confirmed by other studies. The MICRO-HOPE (Microalbuminuria, Cardiovascular and Renal Outcomes Substudy of the Heart Outcomes Prevention Efficacy) trial showed a 24% RR reduction in the incidence of overt nephropathy after 4.5 years of ramipril treatment compared with placebo (6.5% vs. 8.4%, $P = 0.027$).

Treatment with ramipril in patients with chronic renal insufficiency in the REIN (Ramipril Efficacy in Nephropathy) follow-up study was associated with a decrease in progression to dialysis over 36 months (12% vs. 30%, RR: 2.95, 95% CI: 1.13–7.68) [21]. The degree of decline in the glomerular filtration rate per month was decreased significantly (0.10 vs. 0.14 mL/min/1.73m^2, $P = 0.017$). On multivariate analysis, randomization to ramipril treatment was significantly associated with a decreased risk of endstage renal failure after 2 years (24% vs. 40%, $P = 0.04$). This decreased risk remained significant even after adjusting for changes in BP. During a follow-up period of 36–54 months, no patients in the ramipril-treatment group developed endstage renal failure, compared with 30% of patients randomized to placebo plus conventional antihypertensive treatment [21].

Cardiovascular benefits of ACE inhibition have been shown in many clinical trials. In a retrospective analysis of GISSI-3 (Gruppo Italiano per lo Studio Della Sopravvivenza Nell'Infarto Miocardico), early treatment with lisinopril (initiation within 24 hours) after MI was associated with decreased mortality at 6 weeks compared with no therapy (8.7% vs. 12.4%, OR: 0.68, 95% CI: 0.53–0.86) and 6 months (12.9% vs. 16.1%, OR: 0.77, 95% CI: 0.62–0.95) [22]. This was also shown in FACET (Fosinopril versus Amlodipine Cardiovascular Events Randomized Trial), where treatment with fosinopril provided equal BP control as treatment with amlodipine in patients with T2DM. Patients randomized to treatment with fosinopril had a 51% decrease in the risk of a combined endpoint of MI, stroke, or angina requiring hospitalization (14/189 vs. 27/191, $P = 0.03$) compared with those on amlodipine. There were no significant differences in the study's primary endpoint of posttreatment cholesterol levels, HbA1c, or insulin requirements in the two patient groups [23].

At-risk individuals, without left ventricular (LV) dysfunction, were randomized to either placebo or ramipril treatment in the HOPE (Heart Outcomes Prevention Evaluation) trial. Ramipril use was associated with a significant decrease in the composite endpoint of

MI, CVA, or cardiovascular death (14.0 vs. 17.8%, $P < 0.001$). In the ramipril-treated group, there were also significant reductions in the rates of cardiovascular death (6.1% vs. 8.1%, $P < 0.001$); MI (9.9% vs. 12.3%, $P < 0.001$); stroke (3.4% vs. 4.9%, $P < 0.001$); all-cause mortality (10.4% vs. 12.2%, $P = 0.005$); cardiac arrest (0.8% vs. 1.3%, $P < 0.03$); and heart failure (6.4% vs. 7.6%, $P < 0.03$). These improvements were observed in addition to treatment with standard therapies – such as aspirin (or other antiplatelet agent), beta-blockers, and lipid-lowering agents [24].

Diabetic patients represented 38% of the participants in the HOPE trial (3,577 of 9,297 patients), and were the focus of the MICRO-HOPE study. Treatment with ramipril was associated with a significant decrease in the incidence of the primary composite endpoint of MI, CVA, or cardiovascular death compared with placebo (15.3% vs. 19.8%, $P = 0.0004$). Secondary endpoints were also decreased in the ramipril-treated group; these included MI (10.2% vs. 12.9%, $P = 0.01$), cardiovascular death (6.2% vs. 9.7%, $P = 0.0001$), revascularization (14.0% vs. 16.4%, $P = 0.031$), and overt nephropathy (6.5% vs. 8.4%, $P = 0.027$). Ramipril significantly lowered the primary outcome by 25%, even after controlling for the change in BP (95% CI: 12–36, $P = 0.0004$). The SBP and DBP were lowered by an average of 2.4 mm Hg and 1.0 mm Hg, respectively. Microvascular complications of T2DM – combined risk of overt nephropathy, need for dialysis, or retinal laser photocoagulation – were significantly decreased in the group assigned to ACE inhibitor therapy (15.1% vs. 17.6%, $P = 0.036$) [25].

Additionally, ramipril has been shown to attenuate the progression of carotid artery atherosclerosis, as assessed by B-mode carotid ultrasound measurement of carotid intimal medial thickness (IMT). The rate of progression of IMT was 0.0136 mm/year in the ramipril 10 mg/day group, 0.0180 mm/year in the ramipril 2.5 mg/day group, and 0.0217 mm/year in the placebo group ($P = 0.033$) [26]. It is likely that the renin–angiotensin system will remain a very important target in the treatment of patients with atherosclerotic disease.

Side effects

Side effects of ACE inhibitor use range from a dry, irritating cough to angioedema, which may become life threatening. In the MICRO-HOPE study, rates of discontinuation of the study medication were similar in both the active-treatment and placebo groups (33% vs. 34%, respectively). Cough was 3.5-fold more common in the treatment group (7% vs. 2%). Hypotension or dizziness resulted in discontinuation of medication in 2% of the ramipril-treated group and 1% of the placebo group. Angioedema was rare, with 0.3% of the treatment group and 0.1% of the control group reporting an episode. The reported incidence of these side effects was almost identical for the entire HOPE study cohort. No significant adverse outcomes were reported to be due to ACE-inhibitor use [25].

Mild hyperkalemia has been associated with ACE-inhibitor use, with as many as 11% of patients developing the condition. Hyperkalemia is caused by the inhibition of aldosterone by ACE inhibitors, the risk of which is reduced by the concurrent use of loop or thiazide diuretic agents. Once hyperkalemia has been identified, subsequent severe hyperkalemia (serum K^+ >6.0 mEq/L) is rare in those under 70 years of age with normal renal function (serum urea nitrogen <25 mg/dL) [27]. Life-threatening levels of hyperkalemia may develop with concurrent use of spironolactone. For this reason a daily spironolactone dose of 25 mg should not be exceeded [28].

ACE inhibitors have also been linked to renal failure. However, in the ATLAS (Assessment of Treatment with Lisinopril and Survival) trial, only a small percentage of patients with T2DM who were prescribed ACE inhibitors had to discontinue treatment due to hypotension, increasing creatinine levels, or hyperkalemia. In this study, 4.4% of the low-dose (2.5–5.0 mg/day) and 3.2% of the high-dose (32.5–35.0 mg/day) lisinopril groups discontinued ACE-inhibitor use [29].

As first reported in 1983, bilateral renal artery stenosis is associated with acute renal failure after treatment with ACE inhibitors. An increased incidence of acute renal insufficiency was noted in patients with either bilateral renal artery stenosis or a stenotic artery supplying a single kidney. This is due to decreased blood flow to an already hypoperfused kidney [30]. For these reasons, it has been recommended that renal function is established both at baseline and after 2–5 days of ACE-inhibitor therapy [31]. It is reasonable to assess plasma potassium concurrently.

Angiotensin receptor blockers

The renin–angiotensin system is a significant contributor to hypertension. The central messenger or mediator of this system – angiotensin II – is the main stimulus for aldosterone secretion, and controls the mineralocorticoid response to sodium intake and volume load (see **Figure 1**). With decreased sodium intake or volume depletion, the angiotensin II level increases. This stimulates aldosterone secretion, resulting in sodium and water retention. It is possible to block the hypertensive effect of angiotensin II using a competitive ARB. The advantage of treatment with ARBs over ACE inhibitors is the absence of cough and a reduced degree of angioedema. JNC-VI guidelines currently recommend the use of ARBs only if an ACE inhibitor cannot be tolerated [14].

The LIFE (Losartan Intervention for Endpoint Reduction in Hypertension) trial compared losartan with atenolol treatment in 9,193 patients who were 55–80 years old with hypertension and evidence of LV hypertrophy (LVH) on electrocardiogram (ECG). The mean BP at the conclusion of follow-up was 144/81 mm Hg in the losartan group and 145/81 mm Hg in the atenolol group. Losartan use was associated with a significantly lower incidence of the primary composite endpoint of cardiovascular death, MI, or CVA, with a 15% RR reduction (18% vs. 23%, $P = 0.031$). Losartan treatment was associated with accentuated LVH regression on ECG compared with atenolol treatment ($P < 0.0001$). Significant benefit was observed in the primary endpoint of total cardiovascular morbidity and mortality (18% vs. 23%, $P = 0.031$) as well as all-cause mortality (11% vs. 17%, $P = 0.002$). Interestingly, there was also a lower rate of new-onset diabetes in those on the losartan-based regimen (6% vs. 8%, $P = 0.001$) [32,33].

In the RENAAL (Reduction of Endpoints with the Angiotensin II Antagonist Losartan) study, losartan treatment was compared with placebo in patients with T2DM. There was a significant reduction in the risk of reaching the primary endpoint of doubling of baseline creatinine, endstage renal disease, or death in the losartan group (43.5% vs. 47.1%, $P = 0.02$). The rate of first hospitalization for congestive heart failure (CHF) was also lower in the losartan-treated group (11.9% vs. 16.7%, $P = 0.005$). BP was equivalent in the two groups, so the effect of losartan was not attributed to BP control, but rather to angiotensin receptor blockade [34].

The renoprotective effects of ARBs were also shown in IDNT (the Irbesartan Diabetic Nephropathy Trial) where 1,715 hypertensive T2DM patients with nephropathy were randomized to treatment with irbesartan, amlodipine, or placebo. The risk for doubling the serum creatinine was lowest in the irbesartan group (16.9%), and highest in the amlodipine group (25.4%, $P < 0.001$). Endstage renal failure developed in over 20% fewer patients in the irbesartan group compared with the other two groups (14.2% [irbesartan] vs. 18.3% [amlodipine] vs. 17.8% [placebo], $P = 0.07$ for each) [35]. Irbesartan decreases the rate of progression to diabetic nephropathy independent of the BP-lowering effect.

Parving et al. randomized 590 T2DM patients with hypertension and microalbuminuria to irbesartan (300 mg/day or 150 mg/day) or placebo. Over 24 months, 5.2%, 9.7%, and 14.9% of patients developed nephropathy, respectively (hazard ratio 0.30, 95% CI: 0.14–0.61, $P < 0.001$ for the 300 mg irbesartan group vs. placebo) [36].

It should be noted that, despite the beneficial effects of ARBs described above, no studies have yet proven any incremental benefit of ARBs over ACE inhibitors. The use of ARBs among diabetic patients is therefore reserved for those who are intolerant to ACE inhibitors or in combination with another agent.

Beta-blockers

The safety, tolerability, and efficacy of beta-blocker use in patients with T2DM are now well established. Treatment with beta-blockers after MI was shown to have no significant effect on the 6-month readmission rate for diabetic complications in insulin-dependent diabetics over 65 years of age (2.3% vs. 3.5%, $P = 0.06$) compared with patients not receiving beta-blockers. Higher readmission rates were also not observed in those taking oral hypoglycemics (0.8% vs. 1.3%, $P = 0.07$) and in nondiabetic patients (0.04% vs. 0.06%, $P = 0.60$) [37].

In a prospective study by Barnett et al., one third of 150 insulin-treated diabetic subjects were randomized to receive beta-blockers. Episodes of loss of consciousness were experienced by five patients taking beta-blockers, and 10 patients not taking beta-blockers. Given this equal risk, beta-blocker use was concluded to be generally safe in those taking insulin [38].

After uncomplicated MI, beta-blocker use in diabetic patients confers a 36% RR reduction (14.4% vs. 23.9%, 95% CI: 0.57–0.63) for mortality at 2 years, compared with a 40% RR reduction in nondiabetic patients (17.0% vs. 26.6%, 95% CI: 0.60–0.69) [39]. Another study of patients with T2DM and known CAD revealed a 44% decrease in total mortality with beta-blocker use over 3 years (7.8% vs. 14.0%, $P < 0.05$) [40]. The type of beta-blocker used had no significant effect on mortality. However, there may be other differential effects of various medications in this class.

After 24 weeks of therapy in patients with T2DM and hypertension, decrease in BP (–13.1 ± 4.1 vs. –12.1 ± 3.9 mm Hg) and regression of LVH (–10.3 ± 6.4 vs. –10.2 ± 7.2 g/m²) were equal with carvedilol and atenolol treatment; however, this was not true for glycemic control. Plasma glucose and insulin levels were decreased in the carvedilol-treatment group (–5.4 ± 9.0 vs. 3.6 ± 5.4 mg/dL,

$P < 0.001$ and -1.2 ± 1.2 vs. 1.0 ± 1.3 μlU/mL, $P < 0.001$, respectively) compared with the atenolol group. Serum lipids improved with carvedilol treatment: triglyceride (TG) levels decreased (-32 ± 25 vs. 18 ± 31 mg/dL, $P < 0.001$) and high-density lipoprotein (HDL) levels increased (3 ± 3 vs. -2 ± 2 mg/dL, $P < 0.001$) in patients randomized to carvedilol compared with those randomized to atenolol [41].

Many studies have defined the role of carvedilol in the treatment of CHF. Carvedilol is a nonselective beta-blocker, which also has α_1-blocking properties. To date, these studies have not focused on diabetic populations. Packer et al. showed that, over 6 months, treatment with carvedilol was associated with a 65% decreased risk for death (3.2% vs. 7.8%, $P < 0.001$) and a 27% decrease in rehospitalization (14.1% vs. 19.6%, $P = 0.036$) compared with placebo in patients with CHF and an LV ejection fraction (LVEF) of 35% or less [42].

In the MOCHA (Multicenter Oral Carvedilol Heart Failure Assessment) trial, carvedilol treatment was associated with improved survival in patients with CHF and an LVEF of 35% or less. During a 6-month follow-up period, the mortality rate in the placebo group was 15.5%, whereas the mortality rates were 1.1%, 6.7%, and 6.0% in the high-, medium-, and low-dose carvedilol groups, respectively ($P < 0.001$, $P = 0.07$, and $P < 0.05$ vs. placebo) [43].

Beta-blockers also improve the long-term prognosis after MI. A retrospective analysis of patients enrolled in the Göteborg Metoprolol trial showed that initiation of beta-blocker therapy after hospital admission with suspected acute MI had the same benefit in T2DM and nondiabetic patients. The rate of late infarction (during 3 months of follow-up) was reduced from 16.4% to 3.8% in patients with T2DM treated with metoprolol ($P < 0.05$). In nondiabetic patients, the rate was reduced from 7.7% to 5.0% ($P < 0.05$). There was no evidence of intolerance to beta-blockers due to complications of diabetes. The benefits of these drugs, during MI and as long-term prophylaxis, were felt to far outweigh the possible drawbacks [44].

Calcium channel blockers

Calcium channel blockers (CCBs) are used to treat hypertension in a wide variety of patients. The MATH (Modern Approach to the Treatment of Hypertension) trial was performed to establish the safety of the long-acting CCB, nifedipine. In this study, 1,155 patients from 127 centers (including 157 diabetic patients) with mild to moderate hypertension were treated with sustained-release nifedipine for 12 weeks. There was a significantly greater decrease in SBP (-21 ± 15 vs. -17 ± 14 mm Hg, $P = 0.004$) and DBP (-15 ± 7 vs. -13 ± 8 mm Hg, $P = 0.004$) in diabetic compared with nondiabetic patients. No adverse effects on glucose levels, lipids, or renal function were observed with CCB use [45].

In the diabetic cohort of the HOT trial, treatment with the CCB, felodipine, reduced the risk of major cardiovascular events by 51% in the ≤ 80 mm Hg target group compared with the ≤ 90 mm Hg group (11.9 vs. 24.4 events/1,000 patient-years, $P = 0.005$). Cardiovascular mortality was also significantly reduced (3.7 vs. 11.1 events/1,000 patient-years, $P = 0.016$) with felodipine treatment to the lowest DBP goal [16].

The ABCD (Appropriate Blood Pressure Control in Diabetics) trial evaluated the effect of hypertension control on cardiovascular complications in 480 patients with T2DM. The primary endpoint was the effect of intensive (target DBP 75 mm Hg) or moderate (target DBP 80–89 mm Hg) BP control on 24-hour creatinine clearance over 5 years of follow-up. There was no significant difference in the primary endpoint between the nisoldipine and enalapril groups. BP, blood glucose, and lipid concentrations also had similar control, regardless of the antihypertensive agent used. However, the secondary endpoint of fatal and nonfatal MI had a significantly higher incidence in the nisoldipine-treated group (10.6% vs. 2.1%, $P = 0.001$) [46].

CCBs were also evaluated in the Syst-Eur (Systolic Hypertension in Europe) trial, where 492 patients over 60 years of age were randomized to nitrendipine or placebo treatment (10.5% of patients had T2DM). After 2 years, SBP was 9.8 mm Hg lower and DBP was 2.2 mm Hg lower in the nitrendipine-treatment group. Cardiovascular mortality was significantly decreased with active treatment among patients with T2DM (8.3 vs. 27.8 deaths/1,000 patient-years, $P = 0.01$), as was the stroke rate (5 vs. 15 events/1,000 patient-years, $P = 0.02$), and the composite endpoint of all cardiovascular events (22.0 vs. 57.6 events/1,000 patient-years, $P = 0.01$) [47].

Diuretics

ALLHAT (the Antihypertensive and Lipid-Lowering Treatment to Prevent Heart Attack Trial) renewed interest in thiazide-type diuretics as first-line therapeutic agents for hypertension. Chlorthalidone was compared with amlodipine and lisinopril over 6 years – 36% of the 33,357 patients enrolled in this study had T2DM. There was no significant difference in the primary endpoint of fatal CHD or nonfatal MI (chlorthalidone 11.5% vs. amlodipine 11.3% vs. lisinopril 11.4%). All-cause mortality, stroke, and combined CVD were not significantly different between the treatment groups. Heart failure was significantly less common in the chlorthalidone-treated group compared with the amlodipine (7.7% vs. 10.2%, $P < 0.001$) or lisinopril groups (7.7% vs. 8.7%, $P < 0.001$). The ALLHAT authors suggest that thiazide diuretics should remain a first-line treatment for hypertension due to comparable clinical results and lower cost than CCBs or ACE inhibitors [48].

SHEP (the Systolic Hypertension in the Elderly Program) randomized 4,736 patients over the age of 60 years – 583 had T2DM – to chlorthalidone or placebo treatment for isolated systolic hypertension (SBP 160–219 mm Hg and DBP <90 mm Hg). Over 5 years of follow-up, the risk for major cardiovascular events was reduced by 34% with active treatment, in both T2DM (21.4% vs. 31.5%) and nondiabetic patients (13.3% vs. 18.4%). The SHEP authors also strongly recommend consideration of thiazide diuretics as a first-line therapy for systolic hypertension in patients with T2DM [11].

Lipids

Risk

In T2DM patients, the composition of lipoproteins, as well as the level of lipoproteins present in the serum, are linked to the risk for CVD. The diabetic lipid profile is distinctive. Although the LDL level is modestly elevated, there is a greater proportion of small, dense, oxidated LDLs. Furthermore, diabetic patients have an elevated TG level – especially if they are insulin resistant and/or have poor glycemic control – and lower levels of circulating HDLs. T2DM patients with hypercholesterolemia benefit from lipid lowering at least as much as those without T2DM for reduction of the risk of a major cardiovascular event [49].

Therapy goals

NCEP/ATP (the National Cholesterol Education Program Adult Treatment Panel) III has defined the current recommendations for the detection, evaluation, and treatment of hypercholesterolemia in adults. The current goal is to reach a total cholesterol level of <200 mg/dL; levels >240 mg/dL are considered high. The HDL level goal is 40–60 mg/dL, and LDL levels <100 mg/dL are considered optimal and should be the goal in patients with known CHD or diabetes. Non-HDL cholesterol (total cholesterol minus HDL) should be <130 mg/dL.

LDL goals are stratified according to each patient's risk profile. The goal LDL is <130 mg/dL with two risk factor for CHD (non-HDL <160 mg/dL), and <160 mg/dL with 0–1 risk factors (non-HDL <190 mg/dL). Reaching the LDL goal is the primary target of therapy in all patients, regardless of their diabetic status [50].

Major cardiac risk factors include smoking, hypertension requiring medication (or BP >140/90 mm Hg), HDL level <40 mg/dL, family history of premature CAD (first-degree male relative under 55 years

---

Cholesterol

The treatment goal is an LDL level <100 mg/dL

Trial of lifestyle modification for 6–8 weeks

Statins are the drug of choice if diet and exercise are unsuccessful

Consider fibric acid derivatives if the LDL level is 100–129 mg/dL and the HDL level is <40 mg/dL

Niacin should be used with care, if at all, because it increases blood glucose levels

---

Table 2. Treatment of dyslipidemia. Initially, a nonpharmacologic treatment is recommended. Medications can then be added as needed to reach treatment goals. The main target of therapy is low-density lipoproteins (LDLs). HDL: high-density lipoprotein.

old or female relative less than 65 years old), and age greater than 45 years for men or greater than 55 years for women. The number of risk factors present determines the LDL goal of lipid-lowering therapy. HDL and TG goals do not change with increasing numbers of risk factors. It is recommended that secondary causes of dyslipidemia are evaluated in all patients. These include T2DM, hypothyroidism, liver disease, renal insufficiency, and medications (progestin, anabolic steroids, and corticosteroids). Although diet and exercise are the first treatment steps for controlling lipids, adding drug therapy should be considered if the LDL goal is not met after 12 weeks of lifestyle modification. Most people with T2DM and an LDL level >130 mg/dL will need medication as well as lifestyle modification (see **Table 2**) [50].

Statins

Statins inhibit hepatic 3-hydroxy-3-methyl-glutaryl-coenzyme A (HMG-CoA) reductase, which is the rate-limiting step in endogenous cholesterol synthesis. These are currently the lipid-lowering drugs of choice in patients with diabetes due to a favorable LDL:HDL ratio change [49]. The safety of statin use in diabetic patients has been well established.

In one study, simvastatin treatment in T2DM patients resulted in a 38% reduction in LDL levels (from 215 to 113 mg/dL, $P < 0.001$), and a 15% reduction in TGs (from 231 to 196 mg/dL, $P < 0.05$). There were no adverse effects on glucose control or measures of coagulation [51].

The CARE (Cholesterol and Recurrent Events) trial demonstrated the benefit of lowering cholesterol levels after an MI, even in patients with average cholesterol levels. In this study, 4,159 patients – 586 had T2DM – with a history of MI and total cholesterol <240 mg/dL were enrolled and randomized to pravastatin or placebo for 5 years. Among the patients with T2DM, there was a significant reduction in the occurrence of the primary endpoint of a fatal coronary event or MI with pravastatin compared with placebo (29% vs. 37%, $P = 0.05$). Among the entire cohort, pravastatin therapy significantly reduced the rate of nonfatal MI (6.5% vs. 8.3%, $P = 0.02$), coronary bypass surgery (7.5% vs. 10.0%, $P = 0.005$), coronary angioplasty (8.3% vs. 10.5%, $P = 0.01$), and stroke (2.6% vs. 3.8%, $P = 0.03$). There was no difference in all-cause or noncardiac mortality [52].

A post-hoc analysis of 4S (the Scandinavian Simvastatin Survival Study) showed that changes in serum lipids were similar with simvastatin treatment in the 202 subjects with T2DM and the 4,242 nondiabetics. Simvastatin reduced all-cause mortality by 43% in T2DM patients compared with placebo, but this did not reach statistical significance (14.3% vs. 24.7%, $P = 0.087$). However, there were significant decreases in the rates of major CHD events (45.3% vs. 22.9%, $P = 0.002$) and any atherosclerotic event (62.9% vs. 43.8%, $P = 0.018$). A trend towards greater risk reduction was noted in diabetic patients. It was suggested that the diabetic patients had greater absolute clinical benefit from cholesterol lowering because of a higher absolute risk of atherosclerotic events [53].

In an analysis of two secondary prevention trials, pravastatin compared with placebo was shown to significantly decrease the risk of CHD events in patients with T2DM and an LDL level <125 mg/dL (22% vs. 34%, $P = 0.004$). This reduced the risk to the same rate as in nondiabetic patients [54].

In the Heart Protection Study, statin therapy also improved outcomes in patients with normal LDL levels. In this study, 20,536 adults in the UK were randomized to simvastatin (40 mg/day) or placebo for 5 years. The primary outcome of all-cause mortality was significantly decreased in the group taking simvastatin (12.9% vs. 14.7%, $P = 0.0003$). This effect was observed in every subcategory studied, including diabetic patients. There were also significant reductions in coronary death (8.7% vs. 11.8%, $P = 0.0005$), stroke (4.3% vs. 5.7%, $P < 0.0001$), and the need for revascularization (9.1% vs. 11.7%, $P < 0.0001$) [55].

Fibric acid derivatives

The fibric acid derivatives are an alternative therapy in patients who are intolerant to statins. They stimulate lipoprotein lipase activity, which increases hydrolysis of TGs. In VA-HIT (the Veterans Affairs Cooperative Studies Program High-Density Lipoprotein Intervention Trial), 2,531 men with known CHD, an HDL level <40 mg/dL, and an LDL level >140 mg/dL were randomized to gemfibrozil treatment (1200 mg/day) or placebo and followed for 5 years. Gemfibrozil therapy increased HDL levels (34 vs. 32 mg/dL, $P < 0.001$), and decreased TGs (115 vs. 166 mg/dL, $P < 0.001$) and total cholesterol (170 vs. 177 mg/dL, $P < 0.001$). LDL cholesterol was not affected. The primary outcome of the combined incidence of nonfatal MI or death from CHD was significantly reduced in patients with T2DM randomized to gemfibrozil (28% vs. 36%, $P = 0.05$) [56].

The primary prevention of CHD was assessed in the Helsinki Heart Study, which randomized 4,081 men to gemfibrozil (600 mg twice/day) or placebo for 5 years. In the active-treatment group, HDL cholesterol levels were increased (48 vs. 40 mg/dL, $P < 0.01$); there were decreases in LDL cholesterol (157 vs. 171 mg/dL, $P < 0.01$), TGs (98 vs. 205 mg/dL, $P < 0.01$), and total cholesterol (211 vs. 242 mg/dL, $P < 0.01$) [57]. This was associated with a significant reduction in CHD events (27.3 vs. 41.4 events/1,000 patients, $P < 0.02$); however, significant differences were not observed in CHD death or all-cause mortality [58].

DAIS (the Diabetes Atherosclerosis Intervention Study) evaluated the efficacy of micronized fenofibrate in 418 patients with T2DM [59]. This group of diabetic patients had reasonable glycemic control, with a mean HbA1c level of 7.5%, mild lipoprotein abnormalities, and at least one visible coronary lesion. As expected, there was an improvement in lipoprotein levels in the fenofibrate-treatment group compared with placebo. Fenofibrate therapy also resulted in a modest yet significant difference in lesion morphology, as assessed by quantitative coronary angiography. The fenofibrate group had a smaller increase in diameter stenosis (2.11% vs. 3.65%, $P = 0.02$) and a smaller decrease in the minimum lumen diameter (0.06 vs. 0.10 mm, $P = 0.029$) compared with the placebo group. These findings are important given the aggressive nature of disease progression in patients with diabetes.

Niacin

The B-complex vitamin – niacin – decreases free-fatty acid transport to the liver from peripheral tissues, which leads to a decrease in both the synthesis of TGs and the secretion of very low-density lipoproteins (VLDL). Although this is linked to improved lipid profiles, niacin therapy has also been associated with a worsening of glycemic control [60]. Therefore, niacin should only be considered for use in T2DM patients who are intolerant to other lipid-lowering drugs, or those who are unable to reach treatment goals with other therapies.

Blood glucose levels should be closely monitored in patients with T2DM who take niacin [49]. This was addressed in an open-label study of 499 patients who took sustained-release niacin for up to 96 weeks. The baseline fasting glucose level of 96.7 mg/dL was increased by 6.9% with sustained-release niacin therapy ($P < 0.01$). Lipids were improved, with a significant increase in HDL levels (58 vs. 44 mg/dL, $P < 0.01$), and decreases in total cholesterol (246 vs. 273 mg/dL, $P < 0.01$), LDL (163 vs. 198 mg/dL, $P < 0.01$), and TG levels (118 vs. 160 mg/dL, $P < 0.01$) [61]. Niacin therapy decreased total mortality over 15 years of follow-up in the Coronary Drug Project (52.0% vs. 58.2%, $P = 0.004$) [62].

Bile acid sequestrants

These sequestrants bind bile acids in the intestine and increase their excretion in the stool. In a small study of 21 patients with T2DM, cholestyramine reduced total cholesterol (187 vs. 230 mg/dL, $P < 0.001$) and LDL levels (187 vs. 230 mg/dL, $P < 0.001$) compared with placebo. TG levels were increased (189 vs. 176 mg/dL, $P = 0.02$) and glucose levels decreased (116 vs. 136 mg/dL, $P = 0.002$). However, 9.5% of patients stopped taking the drug due to constipation [63]. These drugs are not well received by patients due to gastrointestinal side effects, so their use is limited.

Omega-3 fatty acids

Omega-3 fatty acids are either plant-derived (α-linoleic acid) or marine-derived (eicosapentaenoic acid). Fish – such as tuna, herring, and mackerel – are particularly good sources. In addition to an associated decrease in TG levels, omega-3 fatty acids are linked with other potential cardioprotective effects, including decreased ventricular arrhythmias, decreased inflammation, improved endothelial relaxation, and a mild hypotensive effect [64].

The GISSI-Prevenzione trial randomized 11,323 patients with recent MI (<3 months) to supplementation with: omega-3 fatty acids; vitamin E; a combination of omega-3 fatty acids and vitamin E; or no treatment, in addition to conventional therapy. In addition to a 4.6% decrease in TG levels in the omega-3 group, there were significant reductions in total mortality (8.4% vs. 9.8%, $P < 0.01$), cardiovascular death (5.5% vs. 6.5%, $P < 0.001$), and sudden death (2.0% vs. 2.7%, $P < 0.001$) over 42 months of follow-up compared with the no-treatment group [65].

Current American Heart Association (AHA) recommendations are to include at least two servings of fish high in eicosapentaenoic acid per week, as well as food sources such as walnuts and canola oil, which are high in α-linoleic acid. Supplementation is recommended for those with CAD or hypertriglyceridemia, but only after consultation with a physician [1].

Oral antiplatelet therapy

Risk
Platelet-mediated thrombosis has become a major target for preventing and treating suspected ACS or MI. The effectiveness of antiplatelet therapy is well established for both the primary and secondary treatment of CVD; however, the benefits must be weighed against the increased risk of bleeding that is associated with these medications.

Therapy goals
The benefit of aspirin use has been shown to extend to at least 5 years of treatment. The ADA recommends that all T2DM patients with known macrovascular disease should take aspirin daily. Aspirin therapy should be considered for those over the age of 40 years with T2DM and at least one other risk factor for CVD [15]. Extensive research on the thienopyridine inhibitors has shown a benefit for at least 1 year after an ACS or coronary stenting (see **Table 3**).

Aspirin
Aspirin irreversibly inhibits cyclo-oxygenase in arterial walls and platelets. This action produces an antithrombotic effect by inhibiting the production of thromboxane A_2. Cyclo-oxygenase is nearly completely inhibited within 3–4 days of initiating aspirin treatment of at least 75 mg/day. In situations where it is desirable to attain platelet inhibition more quickly, it is reasonable to treat for a few days with at least 160 mg/day aspirin.

The Antiplatelet Trialists' Collaboration performed a meta-analysis of 142 studies regarding platelet inhibition. In the 49 trials

---

Antiplatelet therapy

Aspirin

75–325 mg/day with documented macrovascular disease

Initiate treatment at age 40 years in T2DM patients with one other risk factor

Consider treatment in T2DM patients between 30–40 years old

Avoid use in those under 21 years due to the risk of Reye's syndrome (a potentially fatal acute encephalopathy with fatty infiltration of the liver)

Clopidogrel

75 mg/day in those who are intolerant to aspirin

Consider long-term daily use in T2DM patients after acute coronary syndromes

---

Table 3. Antiplatelet therapy. Aspirin is the antiplatelet agent of choice and treatment should be continued indefinitely.

comparing aspirin with placebo, there were 45,019 subjects; 22,471 of these were on daily aspirin doses ranging from 30 to 1500 mg (most subjects [99.3%] were on doses $\geq$75 mg/day). A 25% risk reduction (two-tailed $P < 0.00001$) in vascular events (nonfatal MI, nonfatal stroke, or vascular death) was observed with daily aspirin therapy compared with placebo in high-risk patients (those with documented MI, history of stroke, or other vascular disease) [66].

The ETDRS (Early Treatment Diabetic Retinopathy Study) Report 14 examined the effect of treatment with aspirin (650 mg/day) in 3,711 T2DM patients. There was a 9% RR reduction (12.1% vs. 14.9%, $P = 0.24$) in the primary outcome of all-cause mortality during 5 years of follow-up. Aspirin therapy was associated with a significant decrease in the risk of MI compared with placebo (9.1% vs. 12.3%, $P = 0.04$) [67].

Multiple studies, including the HOT trial and a meta-analysis by the Antiplatelet Trialists' Collaboration, have demonstrated the benefits of aspirin therapy, regardless of diabetes status. Medium-dose aspirin (75–325 mg/day) was just as effective as higher doses at decreasing the risk of cardiovascular death, CVA, or nonfatal MI [16,66]. In the HOT study, nonfatal major bleeding was more common in the aspirin-treated group (1.4% vs. 0.75%, $P < 0.001$), but fatal bleeding was equal in the aspirin-treated and placebo groups (0.07% vs. 0.08%) [16].

Thienopyridine inhibitors

The thienopyridine inhibitors (or ADP-binding inhibitors) are a class of drugs that inhibit binding of ADP to platelet receptors. This hinders platelet aggregation via a different pathway than that affected by aspirin. The CAPRIE (Clopidogrel versus Aspirin in Patients at Risk of Ischemic Events) study randomized 19,185 patients with known atherosclerotic disease to treatment with clopidogrel (75 mg/day) or aspirin (325 mg/day). Analysis showed a statistically significant decrease in the primary composite endpoint of vascular death, MI, CVA, and rehospitalization with ischemia (including angina, transient ischemic attack, or limb ischemia) or bleeding in those taking clopidogrel (13.7% vs. 15.1%, $P = 0.011$). There was no difference in all-cause mortality over the 1.6 years of follow-up, but clopidogrel use was associated with a significantly lower incidence of gastrointestinal bleeding (0.7% vs. 1.1%, $P = 0.012$) [68].

The subset of CAPRIE patients with T2DM was analyzed to define the role of thienopyridine inhibitor use in this high-risk group. Of the 3,866 patients with T2DM enrolled in the study, 1,914 were randomized to clopidogrel treatment. The absolute risk reduction with clopidogrel compared with aspirin was larger in this group than in the nondiabetic group (2.1%, $P = 0.042$ vs. 0.9%, $P = 0.096$), but the RR reduction was not statistically different (12.5% vs. 6.1%, $P = 0.361$). In multivariate analysis, clopidogrel use was independently associated with a decrease in the primary composite endpoint [69].

In the CURE (Clopidogrel in Unstable Angina to Prevent Recurrent Events) trial, 12,562 patients (2,840 had T2DM) with ACS, but without ST-segment elevation MI, were randomly assigned to clopidogrel (300 mg once then 75 mg/day) or placebo, in addition to aspirin (75–325 mg/day), for 3–12 months. The first primary endpoint – a composite of cardiovascular death, nonfatal MI, or stroke – occurred less often in the clopidogrel group than in the placebo group (9.3% vs. 11.4%, $P < 0.001$).

The second primary outcome added refractory ischemia to the above, and was also significantly less frequent in the clopidogrel group (16.5% vs. 18.8%, $P < 0.001$). There was an increase in major bleeding with clopidogrel (3.7% vs. 2.7%, $P = 0.001$), but not life-threatening bleeding (2.1% vs. 1.8%, $P = 0.13$). Clopidogrel use was associated with a similar decrease in the incidence of the primary endpoint in diabetic and nondiabetic patients (15% vs. 20%) [70].

Glycoprotein IIb/IIIa inhibitors
GPIIb/IIIa inhibitors hinder platelet aggregation by binding to receptors on the platelet surface that function as adhesion molecules when activated. These medications are used in ACS and during percutaneous coronary intervention. The use of GPIIb/IIIa inhibitors during revascularization procedures in diabetics is discussed in Chapter 7.

Diabetes-specific treatments

Risk
Hyperglycemia is a well-established risk factor for micro- and macrovascular complications of diabetes. UKPDS 35 showed that each 1% increase in the HbA1c level is associated with a 21% increase ($P < 0.0001$) in the incidence of diabetic complications. There was no threshold of risk observed for any endpoint [71].

Intensive glucose control in diabetics has been shown to reduce the risk of cardiovascular events. DCCT (the Diabetes Control and

Complications Trial) showed that intensive blood glucose control decreased the risk of the combined endpoint of major macrovascular events over 6.5 years compared with conventional treatment, although this was not statistically significant (0.49 vs. 0.84 events/100 patient-years, $P = 0.082$). The risk of MI was almost 5-fold higher in the conventional treatment group (0.29 vs. 0.06 events/100 patient-years, $P = 0.065$) [72]. Subjects in DCCT were young, insulin-dependent diabetics; therefore, the applicability of these results to older patients with T2DM has been questioned [73].

Therapy goals

The glucose hypothesis states that hyperglycemia itself is a risk factor for cardiovascular morbidity and mortality. In the EPIC (European Prospective Investigation of Cancer)-Norfolk study, a 28% increased risk for all-cause mortality was observed with each 1% increase in the HbA1c level; this was evident even in the group without T2DM ($P < 0.002$ for the trend) [74].

The DIGAMI (Diabetes Mellitus Insulin Glucose Infusion in Acute Myocardial Infarction) study randomized T2DM patients with a previous MI to treatment with insulin infusion followed by intensive insulin therapy or conventional therapy. Insulin infusion followed by intensive insulin therapy was associated with a significant reduction in 1-year mortality compared with conventional therapy (18.6% vs. 26.1%, $P = 0.027$) [75].

UKPDS 35 analyzed the relationship between hyperglycemia and micro- and macrovascular complications in 4,585 patients with T2DM. The incidence of any endpoint related to diabetes was decreased by 21% with each 1% lowering of the HbA1c level ($P < 0.0001$ for the trend). Lowering the HbA1c level also decreased the individual event rates for all-cause mortality, fatal and nonfatal MI, fatal and nonfatal stroke, and amputation [71].

All of these studies indicate that the therapy goal for T2DM patients should be obtaining euglycemia.

Biguanides

Biguanides lower fasting plasma insulin concentrations by enhancing insulin sensitivity. Peripheral glucose uptake is increased, particularly in the skeletal muscle and intestines, and hepatic glucose output is decreased. This increased glucose utilization produces lactate, which is available as a substrate to sustain hepatic gluconeogenesis and avoid hypoglycemia [76]. HbA1c (9.2% vs. 12.5%, $P < 0.01$), plasma TG (121 vs. 146 mg/dL, $P < 0.01$), and LDL levels (212 vs. 251 mg/dL, $P < 0.05$) have been shown to decrease significantly from baseline with treatment with metformin compared with placebo [77]. UKPDS 24 randomized 2,078 patients with newly diagnosed diabetes to therapy with metformin, a sulfonylurea, or insulin. Those randomized to metformin sustained the least weight gain and had the fewest hypoglycemic events over 6 years of follow-up [78].

In UKPDS 34, metformin treatment was associated with a significant decrease in all-cause mortality (13.5 vs. 20.6 events/1,000 patient-years, $P = 0.011$) and MI (11.0 vs. 18.0 events/1,000 patient-years, $P = 0.01$) compared with diet therapy for T2DM. There was a greater decrease in the absolute risk of all-cause mortality with metformin than with an intensive treatment consisting of insulin or sulfonylureas (7.1% vs. 1.7%, $P = 0.021$). This effect was consistent with equivalent HbA1c level reductions [79].

Thiazolidinediones

The thiazolidinediones (TZDs), a relatively new class of drugs, are insulin sensitizers. Troglitazone (the TZD that has been most thoroughly studied) has been withdrawn from the US market due to rare and unexpectedly severe hepatotoxicity; to date, this has not been observed with other TZDs. Many of the beneficial effects shown with troglitazone may represent class effects common to the other TZDs.

Currently, rosiglitazone and pioglitazone are the TZDs available for the treatment of diabetes. Pioglitazone significantly decreases the fasting blood glucose levels and plasma insulin levels in T2DM patients with pretreatment fasting blood glucose levels between 140–240 mg/dL ($P = 0.001$ and $P = 0.0044$, respectively) [80].

Pioglitazone alone, or in combination with other hypoglycemic agents, is associated with decreases in blood glucose (up to 95 mg/dL) and HbA1c (up to 2.6%) levels. Doses of at least 30 mg/day decrease triglyceride levels by 30–70 mg/dL and increase HDL levels by up to 5 mg/dL. The most common side effects of pioglitazone treatment are weight gain and mild edema [81]. General side effects of TZDs include edema, headache, general body pains, and a flu-like syndrome. Rosiglitazone has also been shown to reduce plasma glucose (by 44 mg/dL, $P < 0.0001$) and HbA1c (by 1.03%, $P < 0.0001$) levels when used in combination with a sulfonylurea [82].

Effects of TZD treatment on cardiac structure and function were evaluated in 154 patients with T2DM randomized to a 48-week treatment with troglitazone or glyburide. Serial echocardiographic analysis revealed an increase in the cardiac index (2.64 vs. 2.36 mL/min/m^2) over baseline in patients treated with troglitazone. This effect was not seen in the glyburide-treated group [83].

In a study by Hirayama and coworkers, troglitazone treatment was associated with improvements in several echocardiographic parameters in normotensive T2DM patients over 6 months. In this patient group, the LV mass index was decreased (136 vs. 152 g/m^2, $P < 0.05$) and diastolic function improved. The deceleration time (192 vs. 214 ms, $P < 0.05$) and isovolumic relaxation time (84 vs. 91.6 ms, $P < 0.05$) were both significantly shortened. None of these effects were noted in patients with hypertension and T2DM [84].

TZDs also have beneficial effects on vascular disease. Troglitazone improves endothelial dysfunction in those with occult T2DM as measured by brachial artery flow, before and after a 5-minute occlusion. In a small, nonrandomized study, blood flow did not increase significantly after occlusion at baseline (224 vs. 204 mL/min). After 4 months of therapy with troglitazone

Thiazolidinediones
Decrease fasting blood glucose levels
Decrease vasomotor activity
Inhibit the progression of early atherosclerotic lesions
Decrease intimal media thickness
Decrease left ventricular mass
Decrease inflammatory cytokine levels

Table 4. The benefits associated with thiazolidinediones.

(400 mg/day), blood flow did increase (450 vs. 188 mL/min, $P < 0.05$) in the active-treatment group [85].

In a placebo-controlled study, troglitazone use was associated with decreased neointimal tissue proliferation, as assessed by 6-month follow-up intravascular ultrasound measurement after percutaneous angioplasty and stenting of coronary atherosclerotic lesions. Lumen areas were equal, immediately postintervention (7.3 vs. 7.4 mm^2), but significantly greater in the TZD-treated group at 6 months (5.3 vs. 3.7 mm^2, $P = 0.0002$) [86,87].

Pioglitazone treatment has been associated with a significant decrease in carotid IMT after 6 months of treatment (–0.084 vs. 0.022 mm, $P < 0.001$) compared with sulfonylurea or diet therapy [88]. The beneficial effects of TZDs are summarized in **Table 4**.

Sulfonylureas

The sulfonylureas are a class of oral hypoglycemic agents whose effect is based upon an increase in endogenous insulin secretion by the β cells of the pancreas. UKPDS 24 compared sulfonylurea, insulin, and metformin treatment in patients with newly diagnosed

T2DM who were unable to control the disease with diet therapy alone. After 6 years of treatment, levels of HbA1c were similar in all three groups. However, two thirds of patients randomized to sulfonylureas required additional therapy with metformin or insulin to control symptoms and fasting blood glucose levels [81].

The sulfonylurea, tolbutamide, was studied by the University Group Diabetes Program in the 1960s. Over 8 years, there was a higher incidence of cardiovascular mortality in the tolbutamide-treated group compared with placebo (19.8% vs. 11.4%, $P = 0.005$) [89]. Increased early mortality has also been shown in patients with T2DM undergoing primary angioplasty for acute MI who are treated with sulfonylureas compared with placebo (24% vs. 11%, $P = 0.02$) [90]. A possible mechanism for this increased cardiovascular mortality is the effect of sulfonylureas on ischemic preconditioning of myocardial tissue. Ischemic preconditioning protects the heart from ischemic insults, and decreases infarct size. Sulfonylureas inhibit potassium efflux through the ATP-sensitive potassium channel (K_{ATP}) in the pancreas. This leads to an increased concentration of intracellular calcium, which results in the release of insulin. However, these same channels are present in the myocardium and coronary vasculature, and are crucial to ischemic preconditioning. Activation of K_{ATP} contributes to vasodilation, which is blunted when the channel is blocked [91].

Prevention of T2DM

Lifestyle modification

The best way to avoid the complications of T2DM is to prevent the disease itself. The Diabetes Prevention Project compared lifestyle intervention – 150 minutes or more of exercise per week and 7% of total body weight loss or more – to pharmacologic treatment of diabetes. Over a 2.8-year follow-up period, change in lifestyle was significantly more effective than metformin or placebo for diabetes prevention. However, those randomized to metformin fared better than those on placebo. When compared to patients on placebo, intense lifestyle modification resulted in a 58% decrease in the incidence of T2DM (11.0 vs. 4.8 cases/100 person-years, $P < 0.001$), whereas a 31% decrease was observed with metformin therapy (7.8 vs. 4.8 cases/100 person-years, $P < 0.001$) [92].

The Physicians' Health Study enrolled 21,271 male physicians in the US and followed them for 5 years. Men who exercised at least once a week had a significantly lower incidence of T2DM than those who exercised less often (2.37 vs. 3.74 cases/1,000 person-years, $P = 0.0003$). This risk reduction was more pronounced in men who exercised at least five times a week; the risk reduction remained significant after adjusting for both age and body-mass index [93].

Medication
Several studies have shown a decreased incidence of new-onset T2DM with medications used to treat other conditions. In the HOPE study, there was a decrease in the development of T2DM in the ramipril-treatment group compared with placebo (2.2% vs. 3.3%, $P < 0.0001$) [24]. In the LIFE trial, losartan was shown to decrease the rate of development of T2DM compared with atenolol (6% vs. 8%, $P = 0.0001$) [32]. Other medications shown to be associated with a lower incidence of T2DM versus placebo include metformin (7.8 vs. 11 cases/100 patient-years, $P < 0.001$) [92], troglitazone (5.4% vs. 12.1%, $P < 0.01$) [94], and pravastatin (RR: 0.70, $P = 0.042$) [95]. Captopril treatment was associated with a lower incidence of T2DM compared with conventional antihypertensive therapy (6.1% vs. 6.9%, $P = 0.039$) [96].

Nontraditional markers of risk

Coronary artery calcification
Coronary artery calcification was recently assessed in the Framingham Offspring Study. Results concluded that diabetics were significantly more likely to have subclinical coronary atherosclerosis than those with normal glucose tolerance. However, more patients with impaired glucose tolerance had atherosclerosis that did not reach statistical significance than controls. A pattern of increasing atherosclerotic burden with increasing glucose

intolerance was evident [97]. The use of coronary calcium scoring by computed tomography is currently under investigation; therefore, its role in risk assessment has yet to be defined.

C-reactive protein

C-reactive protein (CRP), an acute phase reactant protein, is a marker of systemic inflammation. In a sample of 936 men between the ages of 45 and 64 years, a significant relationship was shown between elevated CRP levels and incidence of a first major CHD event. Cox regression analysis resulted in an adjusted hazard rate ratio for CHD events of 1.50 (95% CI: 1.14–1.97) in those with increased CRP levels. Diabetes was associated with higher CRP levels in this study (2.84 vs. 1.58 mg/L, $P = 0.001$) [98].

Elevated CRP levels are also associated with increased mortality in ACS. A substudy of the TIMI (Thrombolysis in Myocardial Infarction) 11 trial showed that CRP levels were significantly higher in patients who died than in survivors (7.2 vs 1.3 mg/dL, $P = 0.0038$). CRP levels greater than 1.55 mg/dL were associated with increased mortality 14 days after ACS [99].

A possible treatment for elevated CRP levels is daily HMG-CoA reductase inhibitor. In the CARE (Cholesterol and Recurrent Events) trial, those with elevated CRP levels who were randomized to receive placebo after an MI had a significantly higher risk of recurrent MI or a fatal coronary event (RR: 2.11, $P = 0.048$) than those randomized to receive pravastatin (RR: 1.29, $P = 0.5$) [100]. In the future, CRP may be useful as a clinical marker of increased risk; however, routine measurement is not currently recommended [101].

Lipoprotein a

Lipoprotein a (LPa), a fraction of total serum lipid, consists of an LDL particle bound to apolipoprotein A by a disulfide bond. Elevated LPa levels have been independently associated with increased rates of CAD and CVD. In a community-based study of 9,936 subjects, CAD rates were significantly higher in those men (35% vs. 20%, $P < 0.001$) and women (40% vs. 14%, $P < 0.001$)

with the highest LPa levels, compared to those with LPa levels in the lowest quartile. Rates of CVD were also significantly higher in those with LPa levels in the highest quartile (men: 12% vs. 8%, $P = 0.008$, women: 21% vs. 8%, $P = 0.013$) [102].

Another study found that LPa was not independently associated with ischemic heart disease; however, it appeared to augment the deleterious effects of other more widely accepted lipid risk factors, such as elevated LDL cholesterol levels and low HDL cholesterol levels [103].

A recent study of 62 patients with T2DM, and 67 first-degree relatives with normal blood glucose levels, did not reveal any significant differences in serum LPa levels between groups, nor were any significant differences observed between diabetic patients and healthy controls (24.6 ± 19.9 vs. 25.8 ± 21.2 mg/dL, and 21.3 ± 20.5 mg/dL) [104].

As LPa is incorporated into atherosclerotic plaques, a direct atherogenic mechanism has been proposed to account for the possible role of this protein in CHD [103]. Measurement of LPa levels is not currently recommended [95].

Homocysteine

High levels of the amino acid, homocysteine, result in endothelial dysfunction and injury, followed by platelet accumulation and thrombus formation. Current strategies to treat elevated homocysteine include replacing deficiencies of folic acid, vitamin B12, and pyridoxine [105]. The homocysteine serum level has been shown to correlate with the risk for death from CHD. In the BUPA (British United Provident Association) study, homocysteine levels were significantly higher in subjects who died from CHD than in control subjects (1.8 vs. 1.6 mg/L, $P < 0.001$) [106].

Another study found that the RR for atherosclerotic vascular disease was significantly higher in those with plasma homocysteine levels in the highest quintile (RR: 2.2, 95% CI: 1.6–2.9) [107].

Multiple regression analysis of 358 men with T2DM showed that the total plasma homocysteine level had a significant correlation with HbA1c ($P < 0.05$) [108]. Measurement of homocysteine levels is not generally recommended for risk assessment, but is considered optional for high-risk patients [95].

Silent myocardial ischemia

Silent myocardial ischemia is an important clinical entity in patients with T2DM. In one study, screening tests revealed evidence of MI (such as Q waves on ECG) in 16% of patients with T2DM for more than 10 years and no other risk factors, or those with T2DM for 5 years and other risk factors for CAD. Silent ischemia, with greater than 50% angiographic stenosis, was found in 21% of men with T2DM. The investigators recommended routine stress testing in all patients with T2DM for 10 years or more [109].

The recently published 2002 American College of Cardiology (ACC) and AHA Exercise Testing Guidelines recommend that asymptomatic patients with T2DM who are planning to begin a vigorous exercise program be given a Class IIa indication [110]. In a T2DM population, the most significant predictor for silent ischemia found on multifactorial analysis was ST-T wave abnormalities on a resting ECG [111].

Patients with diabetic neuropathy are at increased risk for silent ischemia. In one study, asymptomatic events were shown to be more common in patients with cardiovascular autonomic neuropathy, as defined by an abnormal Valsalva ratio (RR-interval shortening of less than 10% noted during the Valsalva maneuver). All patients in this study had evidence of neuropathy with pain, impotence, decreased sensation, decreased deep tendon reflexes, trophic changes, and electrophysiological evidence of sensorimotor neuropathy [112].

Proteinuria

A prospective World Health Organization (WHO) study of over 4,400 diabetic patients correlated proteinuria with mortality in T2DM. There was a positive correlation between heavy proteinuria and cardiovascular mortality (27.9 vs. 9.2 events/1,000 patient-years), renal mortality (15.3 vs. 1.3 events/1,000 patient-years), and all other causes of mortality (16.2 vs. 7.3 events/1,000 patient-years) compared to a group with T2DM, but without proteinuria [113]. BP above the mean predicted a progression from micro- to macroalbuminuria in a 5-year study (RR: 4.2, $P < 0.02$) [114]. DCCT reported that intensive blood glucose control reduced the incidence of microalbuminuria (3.4 vs. 2.2 events/100 person-years, $P < 0.02$) compared with conventional treatment [115].

Smoking

Cigarette smoking has also been implicated as a risk factor for increasing the rate of decline in renal function in patients with T2DM. Smokers were shown to have higher plasma creatinine levels than nonsmokers after 5 years of follow-up (1.78 vs. 1.32 mg/dL, $P = 0.02$); baseline creatinine levels were equivalent (1.05 vs. 1.08 mg/dL) [116]. Smoking cessation should be strongly recommended to any person with T2DM.

Conclusion

T2DM is becoming more prevalent and is associated with a high rate of cardiovascular complications. This places an enormous burden on healthcare delivery systems. Diagnostic and therapeutic modalities for T2DM and CVD are the subject of intensive clinical research. Several nontraditional markers for cardiovascular risk are currently available – including coronary calcium scoring, homocysteine, LPa, and CRP. These may add to the clinical usefulness of traditional markers of risk, such as BP, cholesterol levels, and the presence of T2DM.

Treatment of T2DM, as well as other risk factors, decreases the risk of T2DM-related cardiovascular morbidity and mortality. Adjunctive pharmacotherapy used to treat other conditions – such as hypertension or dyslipidemia – may decrease the risk of complications or of developing T2DM. The treatment chosen for T2DM itself may also have a significant impact on risk. Those providing healthcare to T2DM patients have an opportunity to reduce cardiovascular morbidity and mortality with decision-making based upon evidence in the medical literature.

References

1. McKinlay J, Marceau L. US public health and the 21st century: diabetes mellitus. *Lancet* 2000;356:757–61.

2. Gu K, Cowie CC, Harris MI. Diabetes and decline in heart disease mortality in US adults. *JAMA* 1999;281:1291–7.

3. Stamler J, Vaccaro O, Neaton JD et al. Diabetes, other risk factors, and 12-year cardiovascular mortality for men screened in the Multiple Risk Factor Intervention Trial. *Diabetes Care* 1993;16:434–44.

4. Kuusisto J, Mykkanen L, Pyorala K et al. NIDDM and its metabolic control predict coronary heart disease in elderly subjects. *Diabetes* 1994;43:960–7.

5. Haffner SM, Lehto S, Ronnemaa T et al. Mortality from coronary heart disease in subjects with type 2 diabetes and in nondiabetic subjects with and without prior myocardial infarction. *N Engl J Med* 1998;339:229–34.

6. Stone GW, Moliterno DJ, Bertrand M et al. Impact of clinical syndrome acuity on the differential response to 2 glycoprotein IIb/IIIa inhibitors in patients undergoing coronary stenting. The TARGET Trial. *Circulation* 2002;105:2347–54.

7. Haffner SM. Management of dyslipidemia in adults with diabetes. *Diabetes Care* 1998;21:160–78.

8. George PB, Tobin KJ, Corpus RA et al. Treatment of cardiac risk factors in diabetic patients: How well do we follow the guidelines? *Am Heart J* 2001;142:857–63.

9. Tarnow L, Rossing P, Gall MA et al. Prevalence of arterial hypertension in diabetic patients before and after the JNC-V. *Diabetes Care* 1994;17:1247–51.

10. Burt VL, Whelton P, Roccella E et al. Prevalence of hypertension in the US adult population. Results from the third National Health and Nutrition Examination Survey, 1988-1991. *Hypertension* 1995;25:305–13.

11. Curb JD, Pressel SL, Cutler JA et al. Effect of diuretic-based antihypertensive treatment on cardiovascular disease risk in older diabetic patients with isolated systolic hypertension. Systolic Hypertension in the Elderly Program Cooperative Research Group. *JAMA* 1996;276:1886–92.

12. Adler AI, Stratton IM, Neil HA et al. Association of systolic blood pressure with macrovascular and microvascular complications of type 2 diabetes (UKPDS 36): prospective observational study. *BMJ* 2000;321:412–9.

13. Lievre M, Gueyffier F, Ekbom T et al. Efficacy of diuretics and beta-blockers in diabetic hypertensive patients. Results from a meta-analysis. The INDANA Steering Committee. *Diabetes Care* 2000;23 (Suppl. 2):B65–71.

14. The National Heart, Lung, and Blood Institute (NHLBI) – National Institutes of Health. The sixth report of the Joint National Committee on prevention, detection, evaluation, and treatment of high blood pressure. *Arch Intern Med* 1997;157:2413–46.

15. American Diabetes Association 2002. Standards of medical care for patients with diabetes mellitus. *Diabetes Care* 2002;25 (Suppl. 1):S33–49.

16. Hansson L, Zanchetti A, Carruthers SG et al. Effects of intensive blood-pressure lowering and low-dose aspirin in patients with hypertension: principal results of the Hypertension Optimal Treatment (HOT) randomised trial. HOT Study Group. *Lancet* 1998;351:1755–62.

17. Elliott WJ, Weir DR, Black HR. Cost-effectiveness of the lower treatment goal (of JNC VI) for diabetic hypertensive patients. Joint National Committee on prevention, detection, evaluation, and treatment of high blood pressure. *Arch Intern Med* 2000;160:1277–83.

18. United Kingdom Prospective Diabetes Study Group. Tight blood pressure control and risk of macrovascular and microvascular complications in type 2 diabetes: UKPDS 38. *BMJ* 1998;317:703–13.

19. Unger T. Neurohormonal modulation in cardiovascular disease. *Am Heart J* 2000;139: S2–8.

20. Kasiske BL, Kalil RS, Ma JZ et al. Effect of antihypertensive therapy on the kidney in patients with diabetes: a meta-regression analysis. *Ann Intern Med* 1993;118:129–38.

21. Ruggenenti P, Perna A, Ghererdi G et al. Renal function and requirement for dialysis in chronic nephropathy patients on long-term ramipril: REIN Follow-up Trial. *Lancet* 1998;352:1252–6.

22. Zuanetti G, Latini R, Maggioni AP et al. Effect of the ACE inhibitor lisinopril on mortality in diabetic patients with acute myocardial infarction – data from the GISSI-3 Study. *Circulation* 1997;96:4239–45.

23. Tatti P, Pahor M, Byington RP et al. Outcome results of the Fosinopril Versus Amlodipine Cardiovascular Events Randomized Trial (FACET) in patients with hypertension and NIDDM. *Diabetes Care* 1998;21:597–603.

24. Yusuf S, Sleight P, Pogue J et al. Effects of an angiotensin-converting-enzyme inhibitor, ramipril, on cardiovascular events in high-risk patients. *N Engl J Med* 2000;342:145–53.

25. Heart Outcomes Prevention Evaluation Study Investigators. Effects of ramipril on cardiovascular and microvascular outcomes in people with diabetes mellitus: results of the HOPE Study and MICRO-HOPE Substudy. *Lancet* 2000;355:253–9.

26. Lonn EM, Yusuf S, Dzavik V et al. Effects of ramipril and vitamin E on atherosclerosis. The Study to Evaluate Carotid Ultrasound Changes in Patients Treated With Ramipril and Vitamin E (SECURE). *Circulation* 2001;103:919–25.

27. Reardon LC, Macpherson DS. Hyperkalemia in outpatients using angiotensin-converting enzyme inhibitors. How much should we worry? *Arch Intern Med* 1998;158:26–32.

28. Schepkens H, Vanholder R, Billiouw JM et al. Life-threatening hyperkalemia during combined therapy with angiotensin-converting enzyme inhibitors and spironolactone: an analysis of 25 cases. *Am J Med* 2001;110:438–41.

29. Massie BM, Armstrong PW, Cleland JG et al. Toleration of high doses of angiotensin-converting enzyme inhibitors in patients with chronic heart failure: results from the ATLAS trial. The Assessment of Treatment with Lisinopril and Survival. *Arch Intern Med* 2001;161:165–71.

30. Hricik DE, Browning PJ, Kapelman R et al. Captopril-induced functional renal insufficiency in patients with bilateral renal artery stenosis or renal artery stenosis in a solitary kidney. *N Engl J Med* 1983;308:373–6.

31. Fluck RJ, Raine AE. ACE inhibitors in non-diabetic renal disease. *Br Heart J* 1994;72 (Suppl. 3):S46–51.

32. Dahloff B, Devereux RB, Kjeldsen SE et al. Cardiovascular morbidity and mortality in the losartan intervention for endpoint reduction in hypertension study (LIFE): a randomized trial against atenolol. *Lancet* 2002;359:995–1003.

33. Lindholm LH, Ibsen H, Dahloff B et al. Cardiovascular morbidity and mortality in patients with diabetes in the Losartan Intervention for Endpoint Reduction in Hypertension Study (LIFE): a randomized trial against atenolol. *Lancet* 2002;359:1004–10.

34. Brenner BM, Cooper ME, de Zeeuw D et al. Effects of losartan on renal and cardiovascular outcomes in patients with Type 2 diabetes and nephropathy. *N Engl J Med* 2001;345:861–9.

35. Lewis EJ, Hunsicker LG, Clarke WR et al. Renoprotective effect of the angiotensin-receptor antagonist irbesartan in patients with nephropathy due to type 2 diabetes. *N Engl J Med* 2001;345:851–60.

36. Parving HH, Lehnert H, Brochner-Mortensen J et al. The effect of irbesartan on the development of diabetic nephropathy in patients with type 2 diabetes. *N Engl J Med* 2001;345:870–8.

37. Chen J, Marciniak TA, Radford MJ et al. Beta-blocker therapy for secondary prevention of myocardial Infarction in elderly diabetic patients. Results from the National Cooperative Cardiovascular Project. *J Am Coll Cardiol* 1999;34:1388–94.

38. Barnett AH, Leslie D, Watkins PJ. Can insulin-treated diabetics be given beta-adrenergic blocking drugs? *BMJ* 1980;280:976–8.

39. Gottlieb SS, McCarter RJ, Vogel RA. Effect of beta-blockade on mortality among high-risk and low-risk patients after myocardial infarction. *N Engl J Med* 1998;339:489–97.

40. Jonas M, Reicher-Reiss H, Boyko V et al. Usefulness of beta-blocker therapy in patients with non-insulin-dependent diabetes mellitus and coronary artery disease. *Am J Cardiol* 1996;77:1273–7.

41. Giugliano D, Acampora R, Marfella R et al. Metabolic and cardiovascular effects of carvedilol and atenolol in non-insulin-dependent diabetes mellitus and hypertension. A randomized, controlled trial. *Ann Intern Med* 1997;126:955–9.

42. Packer M, Bristow MR, Cohn JN et al. The effect of carvedilol on morbidity and mortality in patients with chronic heart failure. *N Engl J Med* 1996;334:1349–55.

43. Bristow MR, Gilbert EM, Abraham WT et al. Carvedilol produces dose-related improvements in left ventricular function and survival in subjects with chronic diabetes. *Circulation* 1996;94:2807–16.

44. Malmberg K, Herlitz J, Hjalmarson A et al. Effects of metoprolol on mortality and late infarction in diabetics with suspected acute myocardial infarction. Retrospective data from two large studies. *Eur Heart J* 1989;10:423–8.

45. Tuck ML, Bravo EL, Krakoff LR et al. Endocrine and renal effects of nifedipine gastrointestinal therapeutic system in patients with essential hypertension. Results of a multicenter trial. The Modern Approach to the Treatment of Hypertension Study Group. *Am J Hypertens* 1990;3:333S–341S.

46. Estacio RO, Jeffers BW, Hiatt WR et al. The effect of nisoldipine as compared with enalapril on cardiovascular outcomes in patients with non-insulin-dependent diabetes and hypertension. *N Engl J Med* 1998;338:645–52.

47. Tuomilehto J, Rastenyte D, Birkenhager WH et al. Effects of calcium channel blockade in older patients with diabetes and systolic hypertension. *N Engl J Med* 1999;340:677–84.

48. The ALLHAT Officers. Major outcomes in high-risk hypertensive patients randomized to angiotensin-converting enzyme inhibitor or calcium channel blocker vs. diuretic. The Antihypertensive and Lipid-Lowering Treatment to Prevent Heart Attack Trial (ALLHAT). *JAMA* 2002;288:2981–97.

49. Kreisberg RA. Diabetic Dyslipidemia. *Am J Cardiol* 1998;82:67U–73U.

50. The Third Report of the National Cholesterol Education Program (NCEP) on detection, evaluation, and treatment of high blood cholesterol in adults (Adult Treatment Panel III) Executive Summary. May, 2001.

51. Farrer M, Winocour PH, Evans K et al. Simvastatin in non-insulin-dependent diabetes mellitus: Effect on serum lipids, lipoproteins and haemostatic measures. *Diabetes Res Clin Pract* 1994;23:111–9.

52. Sacks FM, Pfeffer MA, Moye LA et al. The effect of pravastatin in coronary events after myocardial infarction in patients with average cholesterol levels. *N Engl J Med* 1996;335:1001–9.

53. Pyorala K, Pedersen TR, Kjekshus J et al. Cholesterol lowering with simvastatin improves prognosis of diabetic patients with coronary heart disease. *Diabetes Care* 1997;20:614–20.

54. Sacks FM, Tonkin AM, Craven T et al. Coronary heart disease in patients with low LDL-cholesterol. Benefit of pravastatin in diabetics and enhanced role for HDL-cholesterol and triglycerides as risk factors. *Circulation* 2002;105:1424–8.

55. Heart Protection Study Group. MRC/BHF Heart Protection Study of cholesterol lowering with simvastatin in 20536 high-risk individuals: a randomized placebo-controlled trial. *Lancet* 2002;360:7–22.

56. Rubins HB, Robins SJ, Collins D et al. Gemfibrozil for the secondary prevention of coronary heart disease in men with low levels of high-density lipoprotein cholesterol. *N Engl J Med* 1999;341:410–8.

57. Huttunen JK, Manninen V, Manttari M et al. The Helsinki Heart Study: Central Findings and Clinical Implications. *Ann Med* 1991;23:155–9.

58. Frick MH, Elo O, Haapa K et al. Helsinki Heart Study: primary-prevention trial with gemfibrozil in middle-aged men with dyslipidemia. Safety of treatment, changes in risk factors, and incidence of coronary heart disease. *N Engl J Med* 1987;317:1237–45.

59. Effect of fenofibrate on progression of coronary-artery disease in type 2 diabetes: the Diabetes Atherosclerosis Intervention Study, a randomised study. *Lancet* 2001;357: 905–10.

60. Grundy SM, Vega GL, McGovern ME et al. Efficacy, safety, and tolerability of once-daily niacin for the treatment of dyslipidemia associated with type 2 diabetes: results of the assessment of diabetes control and evaluation of the efficacy of niaspan trial. *Arch Intern Med* 2002;162:1568–76.

61. Guyton JR, Goldberg AC, Kreisberg RA et al. Effectiveness of once-nightly dosing of extended-release niacin alone and in combination for hypercholesterolemia. *Am J Cardiol* 1998;82:737–43.

62. Canner PL, Berge KG, Wenger NK et al. Fifteen year mortality in Coronary Drug Project patients long-term benefit with niacin. *J Am Coll Cardiol* 1986;8:1245–55.

63. Garg A, Grundy SM. Cholestyramine therapy for dyslipidemia in non-insulin-dependent diabetes mellitus. A short-term, double-blind, crossover trial. *Ann Intern Med* 1994;121:416–22.

64. Kris-Etherton PM, Harris WS, Appel LJ et al. Fish consumption, fish oil, omega-3 fatty acids, and cardiovascular disease. *Circulation* 2002;106:2747–57.

65. Marchioli R, Barzi F, Bomba E et al. Early protection against sudden death by n-3 polyunsaturated fatty acids after myocardial infarction: Time-course analysis of the results of the Gruppo Italiano per lo Studio della Sopravvivenza nell'Infarto Miocardico (GISSI)-Prevenzione. *Circulation* 2002;105:1897–903.

66. Antiplatelet Trialists' Collaboration. Collaborative overview of randomised trials of antiplatelet therapy – I prevention of death, myocardial infarction, and stroke by prolonged antiplatelet therapy in various categories of patients. *BMJ* 1994;308:81–106.

67. ETDRS Investigators. Aspirin effects on mortality and morbidity in patients with diabetes mellitus. Early treatment diabetic retinopathy study report 14. *JAMA* 1992;268:1292–300.

68. Bhatt DL, Hirsch AT, Ringleb P et al. Reduction in the need for hospitalization for recurrent ischemic events and bleeding with clopidogrel instead of aspirin. *Am Heart J* 2000;140:67–73.

69. Bhatt DL, Marso SP, Hirsch AT et al. Superiority of clopidogrel versus aspirin in patients with a history of diabetes mellitus . *J Am Coll Cardiol* 2000;35:409A.

70. The Clopidogrel in Unstable Angina to Precent Recurrent Events Trial Investigators. Effects of clopidogrel in addition to aspirin in patients with acute coronary syndromes without ST-segment elevation. *N Engl J Med* 2001;345:494–502.

71. Stratton IM, Adler AI, Neil HA et al. Association of glycaemia with macrovascular and microvascular complications of type 2 diabetes (UKPDS 35): prospective observational study. *BMJ* 2000;321:405–12.

72. The DCCT Group. Effect of intensive diabetes management on macrovascular events and risk factors in the Diabetes Control and Complications Trial. *Am J Cardiol* 1995;75:894–903.

73. Vinik AI, Richardson DW. Implications of the diabetes control and complications trial for persons with non-insulin-dependent diabetes mellitus. *South Med J* 1997;90:268–82.

74. Khaw KT, Wareham N, Luben R et al. Glycated haemoglobin, diabetes, and mortality in men in Norfolk cohort of European prospective investigation of cancer and nutrition (EPIC-Norfolk). *BMJ* 2001;322:15–8.

75. Malmberg K, Rydén L, Efendic S et al. Randomized trial of insulin-glucose infusion followed by subcutaneous insulin treatment in diabetic patients with acute myocardial infarction (DIGAMI study): effects on mortality at 1 year. *J Am Coll Cardiol* 1995; 26:57–65.

76. Bailey CJ. Biguanides and NIDDM. *Diabetes Care* 1992;15:755–72.

77. Cusi K, Consoli A, DeFronzo RA. Metabolic effects of metformin on glucose and lactate metabolism in non-insulin dependent diabetes mellitus. *J Clin Endocrin Metab* 1996;81:4059–67.

78. UKPDS Group. UK Prospective Diabetes Study 24: relative efficacy of sulfonylurea, insulin, and metformin therapy in newly diagnosed non-insulin dependent diabetes with primary diet failure followed for six years. *Ann Intern Med* 1998;128:165–75.

79. Turner RC, Holman RR, Stratton IM et al. Effect of intensive blood glucose control with metformin on complications in overweight patients with type 2 diabetes (UKPDS 34). *Lancet* 1998;352:854–65.

80. Patel J, Anderson RJ, Rappaport EB. Rosiglitazone monotherapy improves glycaemic control in patients with type 2 diabetes: a twelve-week, randomized, placebo-controlled study. *Diabetes Obes Metab* 1999;1:165–72.

81. Chilcott J, Tappenden P, Jones Ml et al. A systematic review of the clinical effectiveness of pioglitazone in the treatment of type 2 diabetes mellitus. *Clin Ther* 2001;23:1792–823.

82. Wolffenbuttel BH, Gomis R, Squatrito S et al. Addition of low-dose rosiglitazone to sulphonylurea therapy improves glycaemic control in Type 2 diabetic patients. *Diabet Med* 2000;17:40–7.

83. Ghazzi MN, Perez JE, Antonucci TK et al. Cardiac and glycemic benefits of trogiltazone treatment in NIDDM. *Diabetes* 1997;46:433–9.

84. Hirayama H, Sugano M, Abe N et al. Troglitazone, an antidiabetic drug, improves left ventricular mass and diastolic function in normotensive diabetic patients. *Int J Cardiol* 2001;77:75–9.

85. Avena R, Mitchell ME, Nylen ES et al. Insulin action enhancement normalizes brachial artery vasoactivity in patients with peripheral vascular disease and occult diabetes. *J Vasc Surg* 1998;28:1024–31.

86. Takagi T, Akasaka T, Yamamuro A et al. Troglitazone reduces neointimal tissue proliferation after coronary stent implantation in patients with non-insulin dependent diabetes mellitus: a Serial Intravascular Ultrasound Study. *J Am Coll Cardiol* 2000; 36:1529–35.

87. Minamikawa J, Tanaka S, Yamauchi M et al. Potent inhibitory effect of troglitazone on carotid arterial wall thickness in type 2 diabetes. *J Clin Endocrinol Metab* 1998;83: 1818–20.

88. Koshiyama H, Shimono D, Kuwamura N et al. Inhibitory effect of pioglitazone on carotid arterial wall thickness in type 2 diabetes. *J Clin Endocrinol Metab* 2001; 86:3452–6.

89. Meinert CL, Knatterud GL, Prout TE et al. A study of the effects of hypoglycemic agents in vascular complications in patients with adult-onset diabetes. VI supplementary report on nonfatal events in patients treated with tolbutamide. *Diabetes* 1976;25:1129–53.

90. Garratt KN, Brady PA, Hassinger NL et al. Sulfonylurea drugs increase early mortality after direct angioplasty for acute myocardial infarction. *J Am Coll Cardiol* 1999;33: 119–24.

91. Engler RL, Yellon DM. Sulfonylurea K_{ATP} blockade in type II diabetes and preconditioning in cardiovascular disease. Time for reconsideration. *Circulation* 1996;94:2297–301.

92. Knowler WC, Barrett-Connor E, Fowler SE et al. Reduction in the incidence of type 2 diabetes with lifestyle intervention or metformin. *N Engl J Med* 2002;346:393–403.

93. Manson JE, Nathan DM, Krolewski AS et al. A prospective study of exercise and incidence of diabetes among US male physicians. *JAMA* 1992;268:63–7.

94. Buchanan TA, Xiang AH, Peters RK et al. Preservation of pancreatic β-cell function and prevention of type 2 diabetes by pharmacologic treatment of insulin resistance in high-risk hispanic women. *Diabetes* 2002;51:2796–803.

95. Freeman DJ, Norrie J, Sattar N et al. Pravastatin and the development of diabetes mellitus. Evidence for a protective treatment effect in the West of Scotland Coronary Prevention Study. *Circulation* 2001;103:357–62.

96. Hansson L, Lindholm LH, Niskanen L et al. Effect of angiotensin-converting-enzyme inhibition compared with conventional therapy on morbidity and mortality in hypertension: the Captopril Prevention Project (CAPPP) randomised trial. *Lancet* 1999;353:611–6.

97. Meigs JB, Larson MG, D'Agostino RB et al. Coronary artery calcification in type 2 diabetes and insulin resistance: the Framingham Offspring Study. *Diabetes Care* 2002;25:1313–9.

98. Koenig W, Sund M, Frohlich M et al. C-reactive protein, a sensitive marker of inflammation, predicts future risk of coronary heart disease in initially healthy middle-aged men: Results from the MONICA (Monitoring Trends and Determinants in Cardiovascular Disease) Augsberg Cohort Study, 1984 to 1992. *Circulation* 1999; 99:237–42.

99. Morrow DA, Rifai N, Antman EM et al. C-reactive protein is a potent predictor of mortality independently of and in combination with troponin T in acute coronary syndromes: a TIMI 11A substudy. Thrombolysis in Myocardial Infarction. *J Am Coll Cardiol* 1998;31:1460–5.

100. Ridker PM, Rifai N, Pfeffer MA et al. Inflammation, pravastatin, and the risk of coronary events after myocardial infarction in patients with average cholesterol levels. Cholesterol and Recurrent Events (CARE) Investigators. *Circulation* 1998;98:839–44.

101. Grundy SM, Pasternak R, Greenland P et al. AHA/ACC scientific statement: Assessment of cardiovascular risk by use of multiple-risk-factor assessment equations: a statement for healthcare professionals from the American Heart Association and the American College of Cardiology *J Am Coll Cardiol* 1999;34:1348–59.

102. Nguyen TT, Ellefson RD, Hodge DO et al. Predictive value of electrophoretically detected lipoprotein(a) for coronary heart disease and cerebrovascular disease in a community-based cohort of 9936 men and women. *Circulation* 1997;96:1390–7.

103. Cantin B, Gagnon F, Moorjani S et al. Is lipoprotein(a) an independent risk factor for ischemic heart disease in men? The Quebec Cardiovascular Study. *J Am Coll Cardiol* 1998;31:519–25.

104. Tian H, Han L, Ren Y et al. Lipoprotein(a) level and lipids in type 2 diabetic patients and their normoglycemic first-degree relatives in type 2 diabetic pedigrees. *Diabetes Res Clin Pract* 2003;59:63–9.

105. Welch GN, Loscalzo J. Homocysteine and atherothrombosis. *N Engl J Med* 1998;338:1042–50.

106. Wald NJ, Watt HC, Law MR et al. Homocysteine and ischemic heart disease: Results of a prospective study with implications regarding prevention. *Arch Intern Med* 1998;158:862–7.

107. Graham IM, Daly LE, Refsum HM et al. Plasma homocysteine as a risk factor for vascular disease: The European Concerted Action Project. *JAMA* 1997;277:1775–81.

108. Abdella NA, Mojiminiyi OA, Akanji AO et al. Associations of plasma homocysteine concentration in subjects with type 2 diabetes mellitus. *Acta Diabetol* 2002;39:183–90.

109. Janand-Delenne B, Savin B, Habib G et al. Silent myocardial ischemia in patients with diabetes. *Diabetes Care* 1999;22:1396–400.

110. Gibbons RJ, Balady GJ, Bricker JT et al. ACC/AHA 2002 Guideline Update for Exercise Testing: summary article. A Report of ACC/AHA Task Force on Practice Guidelines (Committee to Update the 1997 Exercise Testing Guidelines). *Circulation* 2002;106:1883–92.

111. The Milan Study on Atherosclerosis and Diabetes Study Group. Prevalence of unrecognized myocardial ischemia and its association with atherosclerotic risk factors in noninsulin-dependent diabetes mellitus. *Am J Cardiol* 1997;79:134–9.

112. Niakan E, Harati Y, Rolak LA et al. Silent myocardial infarction and diabetic cardiovascular autonomic neuropathy. *Arch Intern Med* 1986;146:2229–30.

113. Stephenson JM, Kenny S, Stevens LK et al. Proteinuria and mortality in diabetes: the WHO Multinational Study of Vascular Disease in Diabetes. *Diabet Med* 1995;12:149–55.

114. Microalbuminuria Collaborative Study Group, United Kingdom. Intensive therapy and progression to clinical albuminuria in patients with insulin dependent diabetes mellitus and microalbuminuria. *BMJ* 1995;311:973–7.

115. The Diabetes Control and Complications (DCCT) Research Group. Effect of intensive therapy on the development and progression of diabetic nephropathy in the Diabetes Control and Complications Trial. *Kidney Int* 1995;47:1703–20.

116. Chuahirun T, Wesson DE. Cigarette smoking predicts faster progression of type 2 established diabetic nephropathy despite ACE inhibition. *Am J Kidney Dis* 2002;39:376–82.

5

Diabetic nephropathy

Steven P Marso

Introduction

Nephropathy is an important clinical complication of diabetes, and is associated with increased vascular risk in patients with both type 1 and type 2 diabetes mellitus. It has a relatively high prevalence in the diabetic population, occurring in 20%–30% of patients. According to the US Renal Data System (USRDS), the incidence rates of diabetic endstage renal disease (ESRD) have increased significantly over the last 20 years (see **Figure 1**) [1]. The number of patients in which diabetes was the primary cause of ESRD rose from 33.7% in 1991 to 43.3% in 1999. According to 1999 USRDS data, an additional 20% of patients with ESRD had diabetes as a comorbidity or developed diabetes within 1 year of initiating hemodialysis. Diabetes is the leading cause of ESRD development in the US and Europe.

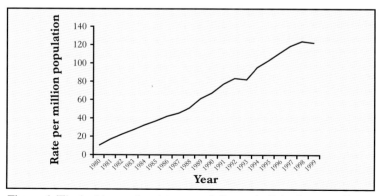

Figure 1. The incidence of endstage renal disease in diabetics according to the US Renal Data System over the last 20 years.

Risk factors for the development of diabetic nephropathy
Duration of diabetes
Genetics: familial clustering
Hypertension
Ethnicity
Dyslipidemia
Smoking
Type 1 diabetes mellitus
Hyperglycemia

Table 1. Risk factors for the development of diabetic nephropathy.

Disease progression

The earliest evidence of diabetic nephropathy is the presence of albuminuria. Initially, microalbuminuria is apparent (low-concentration albuminuria); however, if left untreated, this will progress to overt nephropathy in a substantial portion of diabetic patients in the following 15–20 years. Ultimately, diabetic patients with overt nephropathy will experience a diminution in the glomerular filtration rate (GFR), which may lead to renal failure.

Patients with type 1 and type 2 diabetes have different risks for developing ESRD. Over half (58%) of patients with type 1 diabetes mellitus (T1DM) and nephropathy develop ESRD within 10 years [2]. Without specific interventions, 20% of patients with type 2 diabetes mellitus (T2DM) and nephropathy develop ESRD.

Risk factors for diabetic nephropathy

There are several major risk factors for the development of diabetic nephropathy (see **Table 1**), with the most important of these probably being the duration of diabetes. Although it is commonly believed that patients with T1DM have a greater risk of

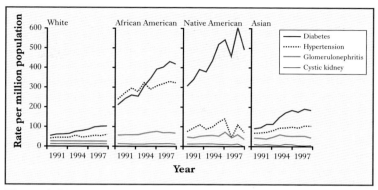

Figure 2. The age- and gender-adjusted rates of endstage renal disease stratified by ethnicity and primary diagnosis.

developing ESRD, the cumulative incidence of diabetic nephropathy is similar for T1DM and T2DM if the duration of diabetes is adjusted for adequately [3–10].

The risk of developing ESRD also varies with ethnic origin. The age- and gender-adjusted rates of ESRD stratified by ethnicity and primary diagnosis are shown in **Figure 2** [1]. In patients in whom diabetes is the primary cause of ESRD, there is a disproportionate risk in African and Native Americans. The Native American population has an annual adjusted incidence rate of ESRD of nearly 600 per million, while the incidence is approximately 100 cases per million in the white population. Other major clinical determinates of diabetic nephropathy are hypertension, hyperglycemia, smoking, dyslipidemia, and genetic factors.

Pathophysiology

Although proteinuria was observed in diabetic patients in the late 18th century, Kimmelstiel and Wilson first described the classical lesions of nodular glomerulosclerosis in the 1930s. The initial histomorphological change in the diabetic kidney is a thickening of the glomerular membrane. Proliferation of the extracellular matrix leads to enlargement of the mesangium. Large, acellular, circular inclusions appear, which have been called Kimmelstiel-Wilson nodules. The molecular underpinnings of diabetic nephropathy are not yet clear; however, hyperglycemia, the formation of advanced glycation endproducts (AGEs), and activation of cytokines may play important roles in the pathophysiology of this condition.

Albuminuria is the clinical hallmark of the development of nephropathy and is associated with increased vascular risk. Initial epidemiological studies demonstrated a heightened risk of developing nephropathy in diabetic patients with evidence of proteinuria. Jarrett et al. and Mogensen et al. reported a high mortality rate in T2DM patients with microalbuminuria [11,12].

Several other studies have linked diabetic nephropathy to increased cardiovascular mortality. In a group of approximately 2,700 patients undergoing percutaneous coronary intervention (PCI), proteinuria was a key predictor of long-term mortality in the diabetic cohort [13]. Patients with diabetes and overt proteinuria had a 2-year mortality rate of 20.3% compared with a 9.1% mortality rate in diabetic patients without proteinuria ($P < 0.001$). A similar heightened risk of mortality in diabetic patients with proteinuria was observed in a coronary artery bypass cohort [14]. Given this well-established link between diabetic nephropathy and vascular disease, it is not unreasonable to screen patients with nephropathy for coronary artery disease (CAD).

Patients with diabetes have a high risk of developing CAD. The American Diabetes Association (ADA) currently recommends stress exercise electrocardiogram (ECG) testing in diabetic patients with typical or atypical cardiac symptoms, such as: an abnormal resting ECG; history of peripheral arterial disease or carotid disease; age >35 years; sedentary lifestyle; beginning an exercise program; and two or more risk factors for CAD – including dyslipidemia, hypertension, smoking, positive family history, and the presence of diabetic nephropathy.

Additionally, patients with diabetes and renal replacement therapy are at exceptionally high risk of developing CAD. According to USRDS data, the presence of both hypertension and diabetes in patients with ESRD greatly intensifies this risk. For example, 55.9% of patients with both diabetes and hypertension, 42.3% of patients with diabetes, 40.3% of patients with hypertension, and 19% of patients with a history of either diabetes or hypertension had concomitant coronary heart disease (CHD). These data exemplify the need for a high degree of clinical suspicion for coronary disease in patients with diabetes and nephropathy, even if they are in the relatively early stages of microalbuminuria or require renal replacement therapy.

Screening for albuminuria

Patients with diabetes should be screened for albuminuria. Given the insidious onset, T2DM patients should be screened for albuminuria at the time of the initial diagnosis. Patients with T1DM should be screened within 5 years of diagnosis.

Microalbuminuria is defined as a urinary albumin excretion (UAE) of 30–300 mg in a 24-hour collection period; albuminuria is defined as a UAE >300 mg/24 hours. The specific definitions are depicted in **Table 2**.

Several screening methods are available:

- spot collection – albumin to creatinine ratio

- 24-hour collection

- 4-hour overnight collection microalbuminuria

- spot urinary dipsticks (requires confirmation with other screening methods)

	Urinary AER (mg/24 hour)	Urinary AER (μg/minute)	Urine albuminuria to creatinine ratio (mg/g)
Normal	<30	<20	<30
Microalbuminuria	30–300	20–200	30–300
Albuminuria	>300	>200	>300

Table 2. Definition of albumin excretion rates (AERs).

Recent hyperglycemia, exercise, febrile illness, marked hypertension, congestive heart failure, and urinary tract infection can all lead to false positive results.

Management of nephropathy

Diabetic nephropathy is undoubtedly a modifiable disease. A great deal of work has been published to date regarding the management of this condition. The primary goal of therapy is to prevent onset and/or delay the progress of the disease. The main facets of therapy are described below.

Glucose management

Numerous studies have established a link between hyperglycemia and the development of nephropathy [15,18]. Furthermore, tight glycemic control modifies the natural history of diabetic nephropathy. DCCT (the Diabetes Control and Complications Trial) studied 1,441 patients with T1DM [19]. Results indicated that intensive therapy (consisting of an external insulin pump, three or more daily insulin injections guided by frequent blood glucose monitoring, or conventional therapy with one or two daily insulin injections) delays the onset and attenuates the progression of diabetic retinopathy, nephropathy, and neuropathy. Over 9 years of follow-up, there was a 34% reduction in the development of microalbuminuria in patients with evidence of proteinuria ($P < 0.04$). In the secondary prevention cohort, intensive therapy was associated with a 43% reduction in the number of patients who progressed to develop microalbuminuria ($P = 0.001$) and a 56% reduction the number of patients who developed albuminuria [19].

UKPDS (the United Kingdom Prospective Diabetes Study) was initiated in 1977 to investigate the effect of intensive glucose control on macro- or microvascular complications in T2DM patients. UKPDS 33 studied 3,867 newly diagnosed T2DM patients [20]. Results indicated that there was a significant reduction in microvascular complications in patients randomized to intensive therapy compared with conventional therapy (similar to the results obtained from DCCT). After 9 years of follow-up, 19.2% of patients in the intensive-therapy group and 25.2% of patients in the conservative-therapy group developed microalbuminuria ($P < 0.001$). Importantly, there was a significant reduction in doubling of the plasma creatinine level in the intensive-treatment cohort (0.7% vs. 1.76%, $P = 0.027$). These landmark trials demonstrated the effectiveness of glycemic control on the development and rate of progression of nephropathy.

Self-monitoring of blood glucose
It is increasingly obvious that diabetic patients should carry out self-monitoring of blood glucose (SMBG) levels and tighten glycemic control. The ADA currently recommends a targeted glycosylated hemoglobin (HgbA1c) level of <7.0% [2]. Both the aggressiveness of glycemic control and the frequency of SMBG need to be individualized. Aggressive glycemic control may not be appropriate in patients with frequent hypoglycemic events, at the extremes of age, and with many comorbidities and a poor life expectancy. Furthermore, the recommended frequency of SMBG depends on a number of factors, including the type of diabetes and the treatment used. For instance, daily SMBG is not unreasonable

in patients taking insulin, and multiple-daily SMBG is commonplace in T1DM patients and pregnant women. The optimal frequency of SMBG has yet to be determined in patients with T2DM. The frequency of SMBG should be adequately individualized to achieve appropriate glycemic goals and detect asymptomatic hypoglycemia.

Management of hypertension

Hypertension remains a prevalent and readily modifiable chronic disease. One in every four Americans (approximately 50 million people) has hypertension [21]. The incidence of hypertension is significantly increased in patients with dyslipidemia, obesity, and hyperinsulinemia; 60% of diabetic patients over the age of 60 years are hypertensive [22]. Concomitant hypertension and diabetes increases the cardiovascular event rate by 2-fold compared with nondiabetics. Furthermore, hypertension in diabetic patients has been linked to several other vascular complications, including nephropathy, retinopathy, and the development of cerebrovascular disease. Unfortunately, many of these vascular perturbations are asymptomatic.

As part of the ARIC (Atherosclerosis Risk in Communities) study, the investigators performed neuropsychological assessments on nearly 11,000 individuals aged 47–70 years old. Asymptomatic subjects underwent two cognitive assessments separated by 6 years. Following multivariate analysis, diabetes and hypertension remained significant correlates of cognitive decline [23]. Middle-aged participants had subclinical, yet readily measurable, deficits in cognitive function over this relatively short period.

Additionally, Kario and colleagues linked the development of asymptomatic lacunar cerebral infarctions to patients with a history of hypertension and hyperinsulinemia. This link persisted following multivariate analysis and was associated with an increase in circulated procoagulants, such as prothrombin fragments 1+2, thrombin–antithrombin complexes, plasminogen activator inhibitor-1, D-dimers, and von Willebrand factor. Furthermore, age and 2-hour insulin area under the curve values were significantly associated with asymptomatic cerebral infarctions [24].

Blood pressure targets

Recognizing the link between hypertension/diabetes and adverse events, numerous expert panels have recommended more stringent blood pressure (BP) targets in patients with diabetes [25–27]. Prior to the availability of substantial clinical data, the Joint National Commission (JNC) recommended a lowering of the target BP in diabetic patients and those with significant renal impairment. JNC-VI recommended a target BP of 130/85 mm Hg, rather than the traditional target of 140/90 mm Hg [27]. This recommendation has since been validated in two large-scale clinical trials [28,29].

The HOT (Hypertension Optimal Treatment) trial and UKPDS 38 implemented multidrug antihypertensive regimens, achieved targeted low BPs, and demonstrated improved outcomes in intensively managed diabetic cohorts [28,29]. The HOT trial randomized 18,790 individuals (1,501 were diabetic) aged 50–80 years with a history of hypertension to a targeted diastolic BP (DBP) of 90 mm Hg, 85 mm Hg, or 80 mm Hg. In the diabetic subset, there was a significant decline in major cardiovascular events in the 80 mm Hg group compared with the 90 mm Hg group; 12.5 cardiovascular events were prevented per 1,000 patient-years (relative risk [RR]: 2.05, 95% confidence interval [CI]: 1.24–3.44, $P = 0.005$). Furthermore, there was a significant reduction in cardiovascular mortality in the 80 mm Hg group; 7.4 lives were saved per 1,000 patients treated (RR: 3.0, 95% CI: 1.28–7.08, $P = 0.016$).

UKPDS 38 compared tight control of BP (<150/85 mm Hg) with less tight control (<180/105 mm Hg). A total of 1,148 hypertensive patients (mean BP at entry 160/94 mm Hg) with T2DM (men and women aged 25–65 years, mean age 56 years) were randomized to either tight control of BP (n = 758) or less tight control (n = 390). Median patient follow-up was for 8.4 years. Tight control of BP with an angiotensin-converting enzyme (ACE) inhibitor (captopril) or beta-blocker (atenolol) achieved a mean BP of 144/87 mm Hg, compared with a mean BP of 154/87 mm Hg in the less tight control group. Tight control reduced the risk of diabetic complications and diabetes-related deaths by 24% and 32%, respectively, compared with less tight control.

Adopting the more stringent JNC-VI guidelines should be both efficacious and economical. Although there will be an increase in the initial cost of implementing the JNC-VI guidelines – in the form of additional pharmacologic agents and the cost of maintaining the program – Elliott and colleagues have demonstrated that money will be saved in the long run [30]. The initial increased cost of targeting a BP to 130/85 mm Hg is offset by a reduction in the development of comorbidities. If JNC-VI guidelines of lower BP targeting rather than the traditional target of 140/90 mm Hg are followed, a 60-year-old diabetic will not only have an increased life expectancy, but also a $1,450 reduction in lifetime medical costs.

Angiotensin-converting enzyme inhibitors
Although many pharmacologic agents have been investigated for the treatment of diabetic-related conditions, ACE inhibitors are first-line agents following acute myocardial infarction (MI) [31] in patients with hypertension [29,32–35] and in the presence of congestive heart failure [36].

Both FACET (Fosinopril versus Amlodipine Cardiovascular Events Trial) and the ABCD (Appropriate Blood Pressure Control in Diabetes) trial randomized T2DM patients to treatment with an ACE inhibitor or a calcium antagonist. Both studies demonstrated a reduction in cardiovascular events in patients randomized to ACE-inhibitor therapy. FACET randomized patients with diabetes and hypertension to fosinopril or amlodipine treatment [36]. Although there was a similar reduction in DBP using both strategies, the fosinopril-treated diabetic cohort had a 50% reduction in cardiovascular event rates, defined as acute MI, stroke, or angina requiring hospitalization. Although diabetic patients were not the primary focus of this trial, these results highlight the importance of ACE inhibitors in this subgroup of patients [35].

The ABCD trial was a prospective, randomized, blinded trial comparing the effects of moderate control of BP (target DBP, 80–89 mm Hg) with intensive control (DBP, 75 mm Hg) on the incidence and progression of diabetic complications. Patients were randomized to either enalapril or nisoldipine [35]. In the 470 hypertensive patients (base-line DBP, ≥90 mm Hg), both enalapril (n = 233) and nisoldipine (n = 237) achieved similar control of BP, blood glucose, and lipid concentrations throughout 5 years of follow-up. However, there was a significantly higher incidence of fatal and nonfatal MI in the nisoldipine group.

ACE inhibitors have also been shown to attenuate the development of nephropathy and other microvascular complications in both T1DM and T2DM patients [37,38]. Ravid et al. evaluated the efficacy of enalapril in normotensive T2DM patients over 5 years. In patients treated with enalapril, albuminuria decreased from a mean value of 143 mg/24 hours to 122 mg/24 hours during the first year. After 5 years, there was a slow increase to 140 mg/24 hours. In the placebo cohort, there was a marked increase in albuminuria from a mean value of 120 mg/24 hours to >300 mg/24 hours. There was approximately a 3 mm Hg decrease in BP, suggesting other potential mechanisms for renoprotection with ACE inhibitors [39].

Angiotensin II increases glomerular pressure, accelerates a decline in renal function, and increases glomerular sclerosis. ACE inhibition – by blocking the effects of angiotensin II – has been shown to reduce proteinuria and albuminuria to a greater extent than other classes of antihypertensive agents. Furthermore, ACE inhibition has been shown to improve epicardial coronary endothelial dysfunction in patients with coronary atherosclerosis [40].

Results from MICRO-HOPE (Microalbuminuria, Cardiovascular, and Renal Outcomes Substudy of the Heart Outcomes Prevention Evaluation) further support these observations. A total of 3,577 patients with a reported history of diabetes were enrolled in the HOPE trial [38,41]. Patients with a history of diabetes were eligible for enrollment if they were over 55 years of age and had another risk factor for heart disease. Patients were excluded if they had an ejection fraction <40% or a history of prior congestive heart failure. Patients were randomized to ramipril or placebo treatment and had a mean follow-up of 4.5 years. There was a 25% reduction in MI, stroke, or cardiovascular death in the ramipril-treated group (P = 0.0004). The mortality rate was 9.7% in placebo-treated patients compared to 6.2% in ramipril-treated patients (P < 0.001). There was also a significant reduction in the rate of MI (12.9% vs. 10.2%, P = 0.01) and stroke (6.1% vs. 4.2%, P = 0.007) in ramipril-treated diabetics.

Angiotensin receptor blockers

Angiotensin receptor blockers (ARBs) may offer a more comprehensive inhibition of the renin–angiotensin system via inhibition of the angiotensin II tissue receptor subtype I (AT_1). Furthermore, ARBs may have improved compliance, as long-term use is associated with a lower rate of chronic cough compared with ACE inhibitors [42].

Initial pilot data suggest that ARBs may have a beneficial effect on renal function. These data have been confirmed by results from four large-scale randomized controlled trials that were recently presented at the American Society for Hypertension 16th Annual Scientific Sessions (see **Table 3**). IDNT (Irbesartan Diabetic Nephropathy Trial) and the RENAAL (Reduction of Endpoints in Non-insulin-dependent Diabetes Mellitus with Angiotensin II Antagonist Losartan) trial evaluated the efficacy of the ARBs, losartan and irbesartan, in patients with T2DM, proteinuria, and elevated creatinine. Both trials demonstrated a significant reduction in the rate of death, ESRD, or doubling of serum creatinine with ARB therapy. In RENAAL, the primary composite endpoint was 43.5% for the losartan-treated group compared with 47.1% for the placebo-treated group ($P = 0.024$). Furthermore, there was a 32% relative reduction in the need for hospitalization secondary to heart failure in the losartan-treated group.

The IRMA II (Irbesartan in Patients with Type II Diabetes and Microalbuminuria) and MARVAL (Microalbuminuria Reduction with Valsartan) trials randomized patients with T2DM, microalbuminuria, and a normal creatinine level to treatment with irbesartan versus placebo (IRMA II) or valsartan versus amlodipine (MARVAL). The primary endpoint in these small controlled trials was the development of frank proteinuria (see **Table 3**). Both trials demonstrated a significant reduction in the development of frank proteinuria with ARB treatment. In the MARVAL trial, albuminuria returned to normal levels in 29.9% of valsartan-treated patients compared with 14.5% of amlodipine-treated patients ($P = 0.001$).

Although ACE inhibitors and ARBs have been shown to be efficacious among patients with diabetes, agents specifically targeted to the diabetic–vascular axis are currently in development. In a modestly sized Phase II clinical trial reported at the American College of Cardiology in 2001, one such agent, ALT-711, was shown to decrease pulse pressure and improve arterial compliance in patients over 50 years old with systolic hypertension. ALT-711 is a thiazolium-based compound that catalytically cleaves AGE-induced crosslinks in the matrix of the vessel wall. These initial results need to be replicated in a large-scale clinical trial, and, if validated, this agent may represent the first in the class of "AGE breakers" to have a beneficial effect on arterial compliance.

Dietary issues

Although there have been no large-scale trials providing compelling human data, small studies suggest that a protein-restricted diet of 0.6 g/kg/day attenuates a fall in GFR. Currently, the ADA recommend a protein intake in patients with overt

Trial	N	Agent	Clinical setting	Primary composite endpoint	RR	P value
RENAAL	1,513	Losartan, placebo	T2DM Proteinuria ↓Creatinine Hypertension (94% of participants)	Death, ESRD, or doubling of creatinine	16%	0.024
IDNT	1,715	Irbesartan, amlodipine, placebo	Hypertension T2DM Proteinuria >900 mg/dL	Death, ESRD, or doubling of creatinine	33%	<0.05
IRMA II	590	Irbesartan, placebo	T2DM Normal creatinine and microalbuminuria UAER 20–200 µg/min	UAER >200 µg/min and >30% baseline	70%	0.0004
MARVAL	332	Valsartan, amlodipine	T2DM Microalbuminuria	UAER		<0.001

Table 3. The effect of angiotensin receptor blockers on renal function in four clinical trials as presented by the American Society of Hypertension 16th Annual Scientific Sessions. ESRD: endstage renal disease; T2DM: type 2 diabetes mellitus; UAER: urinary albumin excretion rate.

nephropathy comparable to the recommended daily allowance of 0.8 g/kg/day for a healthy individual. If the GFR begins to fall, restricting protein intake further – to 0.6 g/kg/day – should be considered. It often becomes necessary to restrict sodium and phosphorous if the GFR continues to fall. If the decrease in the GFR is substantial, referral to a nephrologist adept in the care of such patients is prudent.

Conclusion

Diabetic nephropathy is a common microvascular complication. Without adequate screening and aggressive management, it is typically progressive and often leads to renal failure. A multifaceted clinical strategy is warranted, with specific attention to glycemia and hypertension control. It should be remembered that proteinuria is associated with cardiovascular risk in diabetics.

References

1. System USRD. The epidemic of diabetes mellitus in the ESRD population, 2001. Available at URL: http:www.usrds.org/2001pres/html/talks/usrds_2001_asn_talk_files/frame.htm
2. Standards of medical care for patients with diabetes mellitus. *Diabetes Care* 2003;26 (Suppl. 1):S33–50.
3. Humphrey LL, Ballard DJ, Frohnert PP et al. Chronic renal failure in non-insulin-dependent diabetes mellitus. A population-based study in Rochester, Minnesota. *Ann Intern Med* 1989;111:788–96.
4. Knowler WC, Bennett PH, Hamman RF et al. Diabetes incidence and prevalence in Pima Indians: a 19-fold greater incidence than in Rochester, Minnesota. *Am J Epidemiol* 1978;108:497–505.
5. Nelson RG, Knowler WC, McCance DR et al. Determinants of end-stage renal disease in Pima Indians with type 2 (non-insulin-dependent) diabetes mellitus and proteinuria. *Diabetologia* 1993;36:1087–93.
6. System USRD. USRDS 1994 Annual Data Report. Bethesda, MD: National Institutes of Health, National Institute of Diabetes and Digestive and Kidney Diseases, 1994.
7. Cowie CC, Port FK, Wolfe RA et al. Disparities in incidence of diabetic end-stage renal disease according to race and type of diabetes. *N Engl J Med* 1989;321:1074–9.
8. Nelson RG, Newman JM, Knowler WC et al. Incidence of end-stage renal disease in type 2 (non-insulin-dependent) diabetes mellitus in Pima Indians. *Diabetologia* 1988;31:730–6.
9. Hasslacher C, Ritz E, Wahl P et al. Similar risks of nephropathy in patients with type I or type II diabetes mellitus. *Nephrol Dial Transplant* 1989;4:859–63.
10. Pugh JA, Medina R, Ramirez M. Comparison of the course to end-stage renal disease of type 1 (insulin-dependent) and type 2 (non-insulin-dependent) diabetic nephropathy. *Diabetologia* 1993;36:1094–8.

11. Jarrett RJ, Viberti GC, Argyropoulos A et al. Microalbuminuria predicts mortality in non-insulin-dependent diabetics. *Diabet Med* 1984;1:17–9.

12. Mogensen CE. Microalbuminuria predicts clinical proteinuria and early mortality in maturity-onset diabetes. *N Engl J Med* 1984;310:356–60.

13. Marso SP, Ellis SG, Tuzcu M et al. The importance of proteinuria as a determinant of mortality following percutaneous coronary revascularization in diabetics. *J Am Coll Cardiol* 1999;33:1269–77.

14. Marso SP, Ellis SG, Gurm HS et al. Proteinuria is a key determinant of death in patients with diabetes after isolated coronary artery bypass grafting. *Am Heart J* 2000;139:939–44.

15. Klein R, Klein BE, Moss SE. The incidence of gross proteinuria in people with insulin-dependent diabetes mellitus. *Arch Intern Med* 1991;151:1344–8.

16. Nelson RG, Knowler WC, Pettitt DJ et al. Incidence and determinants of elevated urinary albumin excretion in Pima Indians with NIDDM. *Diabetes Care* 1995;18:182–7.

17. Kunzelman CL, Knowler WC, Pettitt DJ et al. Incidence of proteinuria in type 2 diabetes mellitus in the Pima Indians. *Kidney Int* 1989;35:681–7.

18. Coonrod BA, Ellis D, Becker DJ et al. Predictors of microalbuminuria in individuals with IDDM. Pittsburgh Epidemiology of Diabetes Complications Study. *Diabetes Care* 1993;16:1376–83.

19. The Diabetes Control and Complications Trial Research Group. The effect of intensive treatment of diabetes on the development and progression of long-term complications in insulin-dependent diabetes mellitus. *N Engl J Med* 1993;329:977–86.

20. UK Prospective Diabetes Study (UKPDS) Group. Intensive blood-glucose control with sulphonylureas or insulin compared with conventional treatment and risk of complications in patients with type 2 diabetes (UKPDS 33). *Lancet* 1998;352:837–53.

21. National High Blood Pressure Education Program Working Group report on primary prevention of hypertension. *Arch Intern Med* 1993;153:186–208.

22. Haffner SM, Ferrannini E, Hazuda HP et al. Clustering of cardiovascular risk factors in confirmed prehypertensive individuals. *Hypertension* 1992;20:38–45.

23. Knopman D, Boland LL, Mosley T et al. Cardiovascular risk factors and cognitive decline in middle-aged adults. *Neurology* 2001;56:42–8.

24. Kario K, Matsuo T, Kobayashi H et al. Hyperinsulinemia and hemostatic abnormalities are associated with silent lacunar infarcts in elderly hypetensive patients. *J Am Coll Cardiol* 2001;37:871–7.

25. National High Blood Pressure Education Program Working Group Report on Hypertension in the Elderly. National High Blood Pressure Education Program Working Group. *Hypertension* 1994;23:275–85.

26. Jacobson HR, Striker GE. Report on a workshop to develop management recommendations for the prevention of progression in chronic renal disease. *Am J Kidney Dis* 1995;25:103–6.

27. The sixth report of the Joint National Committee on prevention, detection, evaluation, and treatment of high blood pressure. *Arch Intern Med* 1997;157:2413–46.

28. Hansson L, Zanchetti A, Carruthers SG et al. Effects of intensive blood-pressure lowering and low-dose aspirin in patients with hypertension: principal results of the Hypertension Optimal Treatment (HOT) randomised trial. HOT Study Group. *Lancet* 1998;351:1755–62.

29. UK Prospective Diabetes Study Group. Tight blood pressure control and risk of macrovascular and microvascular complications in type 2 diabetes. UKPDS 38. *BMJ* 1998;317:703–13.

30. Elliott WJ, Weir DR, Black HR. Cost-effectiveness of the lower treatment goal (of JNC VI) for diabetic hypertensive patients. Joint National Committee on Prevention, Detection, Evaluation, and Treatment of High Blood Pressure. *Arch Intern Med* 2000;160:1277–83.

31. Zuanetti G, Latini R, Maggioni AP et al. Effect of the ACE inhibitor lisinopril on mortality in diabetic patients with acute myocardial infarction: data from the GISSI-3 study. *Circulation* 1997;96:4239–45.

32. Hansson L, Lindholm LH, Niskanen L et al. Effect of angiotensin-converting-enzyme inhibition compared with conventional therapy on cardiovascular morbidity and mortality in hypertension: the Captopril Prevention Project (CAPPP) randomised trial. *Lancet* 1999;353:611–6.

33. UK Prospective Diabetes Study Group. Efficacy of atenolol and captopril in reducing risk of macrovascular and microvascular complications in type 2 diabetes: UKPDS 39. *BMJ* 1998;317:713–20.

34. Tatti P, Pahor M, Byington RP et al. Outcome results of the Fosinopril Versus Amlodipine Cardiovascular Events Randomized Trial (FACET) in patients with hypertension and NIDDM. *Diabetes Care* 1998;21:597–603.

35. Estacio RO, Jeffers BW, Hiatt WR et al. The effect of nisoldipine as compared with enalapril on cardiovascular outcomes in patients with non-insulin-dependent diabetes and hypertension. *N Engl J Med* 1998;338:645–52.

36. Shindler DM, Kostis JB, Yusuf S et al. Diabetes mellitus, a predictor of morbidity and mortality in the Studies of Left Ventricular Dysfunction (SOLVD) Trials and Registry. *Am J Cardiol* 1996;77:1017–20.

37. UK Prospective Diabetes Study Group. Efficacy of atenolol and captopril in reducing risk of macrovascular and microvascular complications in type 2 diabetes: UKPDS 39. *BMJ* 1998;317:713–20.

38. Chaturvedi N, Sjolie AK, Stephenson JM et al. Effect of lisinopril on progression of retinopathy in normotensive people with type 1 diabetes. The EUCLID Study Group. EURODIAB Controlled Trial of Lisinopril in Insulin-Dependent Diabetes Mellitus. *Lancet* 1998;351:28–31.

39. Ravid M, Savin H, Jutrin I et al. Long-term stabilizing effect of angiotensin-converting enzyme inhibition on plasma creatinine and on proteinuria in normotensive type II diabetic patients. *Ann Intern Med* 1993;118:577–81.

40. Mancini GB, Henry GC, Macaya C et al. Angiotensin-converting enzyme inhibition with quinapril improves endothelial vasomotor dysfunction in patients with coronary artery disease. The TREND (Trial on Reversing Endothelial Dysfunction) Study. *Circulation* 1996;94:258–65.

41. Heart Outcomes Prevention Evaluation Study Investigators. Effects of ramipril on cardiovascular and microvascular outcomes in people with diabetes mellitus: results of the HOPE study and MICRO-HOPE substudy. *Lancet* 2000;355:253–9.

42. Larochelle P, Flack JM, Marbury TC et al. Effects and tolerability of irbesartan versus enalapril in patients with severe hypertension. Irbesartan Multicenter Investigators. *Am J Cardiol* 1997;80:1613–5.

Ischemic coronary syndromes

Benjamin H Trichon & Matthew T Roe

Introduction

Patients with diabetes mellitus have a 2- to 4-fold increased risk of developing coronary artery disease (CAD), and ischemic heart disease is the most common cause of death in this population (see **Figure 1**) [1]. Furthermore, patients with both CAD and diabetes have an increased risk of developing an acute coronary syndrome (ACS) and a higher death rate after suffering an acute myocardial infarction (MI) [2]. This chapter will focus on the clinical presentation of ACS – including non-ST-segment elevation ACS (NSTE-ACS) and acute ST-elevation MI (STEMI) – in patients with diabetes, and review the relative benefits of different therapies for these syndromes.

Pathophysiology of ACS in patients with diabetes

The diabetic state is characterized by vascular endothelial dysfunction and accelerated development of atherosclerosis. Hyperglycemia inhibits the activity of endothelial nitric oxide synthase (eNOS), reducing the production of NO and impairing endothelium-dependent vasodilation. Consequently, the production of reactive oxygen species – especially the superoxide anion (O^{2-}) – is increased, further inhibiting the action of eNOS.

The production of vasoconstrictive agents – namely endothelin-I and angiotensin II – and the activity of inflammatory lymphocytic infiltration in atherosclerotic plaques are higher in diabetic patients [3]. Elevated levels of cytokines and matrix metalloproteinases in

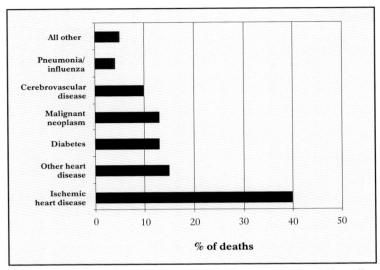

Figure 1. Causes of death in patients with diabetes, based on US studies. Adapted with permission from Geiss LS, Herman WH, Smith PJ. National Diabetes Data Group. *Diabetes in America*. Bethesda, MD: National Institutes of Health, National Institute of Diabetes and Digestive and Kidney Diseases, 1995:233–57.

diabetics lead to a decrease in the synthesis and an increase in the breakdown of collagen in the fibrous cap of the atherosclerotic plaque [3]. All of these factors combine to reduce the mechanical stability of the plaque's fibrous cap. Therefore, the cap is more susceptible to plaque rupture and the subsequent formation of an overlying intracoronary thrombus; the result is the clinical manifestations of ACS.

Abnormalities of platelet function are also central to the increased risk of thrombotic events in patients with diabetes (see **Table 1**) compared with those of nondiabetics. Platelets in diabetics are larger, have a greater concentration of glycoprotein (GP)IIb/IIIa surface receptors, and tend to aggregate more aggressively when stimulated [4]. *In vivo* studies in diabetic patients have demonstrated increased shear-induced platelet adhesion and aggregation, augmented

Characteristic	Effect
Fibrinogen	↑
Plasminogen activator inhibitor-1	↑
Antithrombin III	↓
Protein C and protein S	↓
Factors VII and VIII	↑
Vascular cell adhesion molecule-1	↑
Platelet adhesion	↑
Platelet aggregation	↑
Platelet nitric oxide production	↓
Platelet prostacyclin production	↑
Glycation of platelet proteins	↑

Table 1. Abnormalities of platelet function and coagulation in diabetes mellitus. ↑: increased; ↓: decreased. Adapted with permission from Kirpichnikov D, Sowers JR. Diabetes mellitus and diabetes-associated vascular disease. *Trends Endocrinol Metab* 2001;12:225–30.

synthesis of proaggregating thromboxanes, and a high percentage of platelets circulating in the activated state [5].

Effect of diabetes on the clinical presentation of ACS

Patients with diabetes may have mild or atypical symptoms and signs accompanying an ACS, presumably as a consequence of underlying autonomic and sensory neuropathies. Autonomic neuropathy can impair angina recognition. Atypical ischemic symptoms – including dyspnea, nausea, vomiting, unexplained fatigue, diaphoresis, or disturbances in glycemic control – may predominate the clinical presentation of ACS in diabetic patients.

The frequency of silent myocardial ischemia and MI is high among patients with diabetes. In a cohort of patients undergoing treadmill testing, over 60% of those with silent ischemia had diabetes, and all had underlying autonomic nervous system abnormalities despite the absence of overt vascular complications of diabetes [6]. Additionally, diabetes is often associated with abnormalities of gastric emptying that may lead to frequent noncardiac chest pain syndromes.

In many patients with diabetes, the impaired sensation of ischemic chest discomfort appears to contribute to late presentation of an ACS for medical attention, and subsequent delay in initiation of therapy. In the GUSTO (Global Utilization of Streptokinase and Tissue Plasminogen Activator for Occluded Coronary Arteries)-I trial, patients with diabetes suffering from STEMI presented, on average, about 15 minutes later for treatment than nondiabetic patients [7]. In a pooled analysis of almost 70,000 patients receiving fibrinolytic therapy, the FTT (Fibrinolytic Therapy Trialists') collaborative group found that STEMI-related mortality was 1% higher for every 1-hour delay in treatment from the time of presentation [8]. A similar decremental benefit is observed with delays in primary percutaneous coronary intervention (PCI) for STEMI [9]. This time-dependent benefit of primary reperfusion therapy in the setting of STEMI warrants continued education of patients with diabetes on the importance of early presentation and the potential atypical clinical manifestations of myocardial ischemia that may occur [10].

Electrocardiogram (ECG) findings in diabetic patients presenting with suspected ACS should be interpreted with care. The use of certain oral hypoglycemic medications can produce ECG alterations that may reduce the sensitivity for detecting the characteristic changes associated with myocardial ischemia. Several animal studies suggest that sulfonylurea drugs are associated with a reduced amplitude of ST-segment elevation and T-wave peaking during the early phases of acute myocardial ischemia [11]. Other nonspecific repolarization abnormalities may also be associated with the use of these medications [12]. Because of these potential confounding effects on the ECG, and the high pretest probability of

CAD, physicians and other healthcare providers should maintain a high index of suspicion for ACS when patients with diabetes present with typical or atypical chest pain symptoms and equivocal ECG findings.

Reperfusion therapy for STEMI

Clinical outcomes after fibrinolysis

The results from the major fibrinolytic trials provide an insight into the influence of diabetes on the clinical outcomes of patients suffering a STEMI and the relative efficacy of fibrinolysis in this patient population. In the GUSTO-I trial, which evaluated fibrinolytic therapy in over 40,000 patients with STEMI, 30-day mortality was 10.5% among the 5,944 patients with diabetes compared with 6.2% in nondiabetics [7]. Mortality rates at 1 year were approximately 60% higher in diabetics compared with nondiabetics (14.5% vs. 8.9%; $P = 0.0001$), with the highest mortality rate being observed in diabetic patients who were treated with insulin (12.5% vs. 9.7% in those not receiving insulin, $P < 0.001$) (see **Figure 2**).

The TAMI (Thrombolysis and Angioplasty in Myocardial Infarction) study also reported inferior outcomes in diabetic patients [13]. In the FTT collaborative pooled analysis of data from several large fibrinolytic trials, patients with diabetes receiving fibrinolytic therapy had an almost 2-fold higher rate of mortality at 30 days than nondiabetic patients (13.6% vs. 8.7%) [8]. Despite this higher event rate, the use of fibrinolysis was associated with a larger absolute reduction in mortality in diabetic patients compared with nondiabetic patients (37 lives saved per 1,000 patients with diabetes compared with 15 lives saved per 1,000 patients without diabetes) [8].

More recent studies with new pharmacologic reperfusion strategies, utilizing bolus fibrinolytic agents – such as reteplase and tenecteplase – and combinations of reduced-dose fibrinolytic agents and GPIIb/IIIa inhibitors, have also evaluated the relative

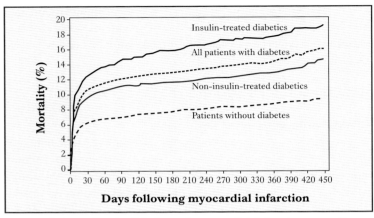

Figure 2. Mortality in ST-elevated myocardial infarction according to diabetes treatment. Adapted with permission from Mak KH, Moliterno DJ, Granger CB et al. Influence of diabetes mellitus on clinical outcome in the thrombolytic era of acute myocardial infarction. GUSTO-I Investigators. Global Utilization of Streptokinase and Tissue Plasminogen Activator for Occluded Coronary Arteries. *J Am Coll Cardiol* 1997;30:171–9.

treatment effects in patients with and without diabetes [14–16]. In the GUSTO-V trial, 16,588 participants were randomized to full-dose reteplase or half-dose reteplase plus abciximab. Of these, 16% had diabetes. Diabetic patients receiving half-dose reteplase plus abciximab had a higher 30-day mortality than nondiabetic patients (8.2% vs. 5.0%), and a similar modest relative reduction in 30-day mortality to that observed in the overall study population [16]. Diabetics receiving full-dose reteplase also had higher 30-day mortality rates than nondiabetics (8.8% vs. 5.3%).

Use of fibrinolytics in patients with diabetes

Despite the greater absolute benefit of reperfusion therapy among diabetics, patients with diabetes are less likely to receive fibrinolytics than nondiabetics. In the SAVE (Survival and Ventricular Enlargement) study, over 67% of enrolled patients with STEMI did not receive fibrinolytic therapy; the presence of diabetes was an independent predictor of the non-use of fibrinolytics (see **Figure 3**) [17].

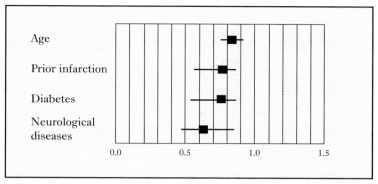

Figure 3. Negative predictors for the use of fibrinolysis in the SAVE trial. Patients with diabetes were less likely to receive fibrinolytic therapy than nondiabetics. Values less than 1 illustrate the odds ratio of receiving fibrinolytics. Adapted with permission from Mak KH, Topol EJ. Emerging concepts in the management of acute myocardial infarction in patients with diabetes mellitus. *J Am Coll Cardiol* 2000;35:563–8.

The low use of fibrinolytics in patients with diabetes was also reported in an observational analysis from NRMI (National Registry of Myocardial Infarction)-2. In this multivariate analysis, the presence of diabetes was an independent predictor for the non-use of reperfusion therapy (odds ratio [OR]: 0.67, 95% confidence interval [CI]: 0.52–0.87) [18]. Additional reports of nationwide practices in France and the UK have found that eligible patients with STEMI and diabetes were significantly less likely to receive primary reperfusion therapy than nondiabetic patients [19,20].

Concern about higher complication rates in diabetic patients should not preclude the use of fibrinolytic therapy in eligible patients with diabetes and STEMI. In the GUSTO-I trial, patients with diabetes had only a small increase in moderate bleeding complications after fibrinolysis compared with nondiabetic patients (13% vs. 11%), and no increase in the risk of major bleeding events was evident. The risk of intracranial hemorrhage in GUSTO-I was also similar in patients with and without diabetes (0.6% vs. 0.7%) [7]. In addition, experience from GUSTO-I suggests that concern over the risk of intraocular hemorrhage should not preclude the use of fibrinolytic agents in appropriate patients with diabetes suffering from STEMI [21].

Primary percutaneous coronary intervention

Primary percutaneous transluminal coronary angioplasty (PTCA) reduces the rates of death, reinfarction, and stroke compared with fibrinolytic therapy for the treatment of STEMI [22]. This strategy has rarely been studied specifically in patients with diabetes, so data regarding procedural success and long-term outcomes are derived primarily from subanalyses of large clinical trials.

The GUSTO-IIb primary angioplasty substudy analyzed the relative benefits of pharmacologic and mechanical reperfusion strategies among 1,138 patients with STEMI randomized to primary PTCA or accelerated tissue-type plasminogen activator (tPA) [23]. Patients with diabetes (16% of the total population) had higher risk baseline clinical characteristics and more extensive coronary disease than nondiabetic patients. The rate of the primary endpoint – death, reinfarction, or disabling stroke – at 30 days was more frequent among diabetic patients treated with primary PTCA than nondiabetic patients (11.1% vs. 9.3%). However, both diabetic patients (OR: 0.70, 95% CI: 0.29–1.72) and nondiabetic patients (OR: 0.62, 95% CI: 0.41–0.96) had similar improved outcomes at 30 days with primary PTCA compared with accelerated tPA.

In a combined analysis of two large primary PTCA trials – GUSTO IIb and RAPPORT (ReoPro and Primary PTCA Organization and Randomized Trial) – the presence of diabetes did not independently predict death or reinfarction at 30 days [24]. Similarly, the presence of diabetes did not independently predict adverse in-hospital and 6-month outcomes in a subgroup analysis of the first PAMI (Primary Angioplasty in Myocardial Infarction) trial, which compared PTCA with tPA [25]. However, Thomas et al. demonstrated a 3-fold increase in the risk of long-term mortality in diabetic patients participating in a trial comparing streptokinase (SK) treatment with primary PTCA [26]. Thus, primary PTCA appears to provide equal benefit to diabetic and nondiabetic patients, and the increased risk of adverse outcomes commonly observed in diabetic patients after STEMI may be somewhat mitigated by mechanical reperfusion strategies.

Stents and GPIIb/IIIa inhibitors

The use of stents and platelet GPIIb/IIIa inhibitors in conjunction with primary PTCA reduces the risk of recurrent ischemia and improves clinical outcomes after STEMI [27]. Several trials utilizing stents and GPIIb/IIIa inhibitors have included significant numbers of patients with diabetes. The CADILLAC (Controlled Abciximab and Device Investigation to Lower Late Angioplasty Complications) trial randomized eligible patients with STEMI to one of four primary reperfusion strategies: PTCA alone; PTCA plus the GPIIb/IIIa inhibitor, abciximab; stenting alone; or stenting plus abciximab [28]. Diabetics accounted for 16.6% of the total 2,082 study participants, and they received a similar magnitude of benefit with stenting and abciximab as the overall study population (OR: 0.56, 95% CI: 0.32–0.97 [diabetic]; OR: 0.54, 95% CI: 0.42–0.69 [total population]).

In the ADMIRAL (Abciximab before Direct Angioplasty and Stenting in Myocardial Infarction Regarding Acute and Long-term Follow-up) trial, patients with STEMI undergoing primary stenting were randomized to abciximab or placebo. Patients with diabetes had a greater absolute reduction in the rate of death, MI, or urgent revascularization at 30 days compared with the total study population (absolute risk reduction [ARR]: 13.9% [diabetics] vs. 8.0% [total population]) [29]. Thus, patients with diabetes who present with STEMI may derive particular benefit from a reperfusion strategy that includes primary stenting and GPIIb/IIIa inhibition.

Despite these encouraging results, the presence of diabetes may increase the risk of early complications after primary PCI. In a cohort of 104 consecutive patients undergoing primary stenting for STEMI, Silva et al. demonstrated that the only independent predictors of stent thrombosis were diabetes and tobacco use [30]. This finding may reflect the increased platelet activation and aggregation in patients with diabetes. This preliminary evidence suggests that diabetes may be an important risk factor for stent thrombosis, in addition to its established role in the development of in-stent restenosis following elective PCI [5].

Early invasive management for NSTE-ACS

Patients hospitalized with unstable angina or NSTEMI (collectively known as NSTE-ACS) can be managed with an "early conservative" strategy, characterized by: medical stabilization; noninvasive risk stratification; and coronary angiography, but only if recurrent ischemia develops. Alternatively, if needed, an "early invasive" strategy can be employed with routine angiography and revascularization within 48 hours of admission in all patients. These two approaches have been compared in several randomized controlled trials, but have not been studied specifically in patients with diabetes [31,32].

The FRISC (Fragmin and Fast Revascularization during Instability in Coronary Artery Disease)-II study randomly assigned 2,457 patients with NSTE-ACS to an early invasive or early conservative management strategy [31]. Of the patients enrolled in the study, 299 (12%) had diabetes. The absolute benefit of the early invasive strategy was greater in diabetic than nondiabetic patients (ARR: 6.2% vs. 2.3%). The superiority of the early invasive approach in diabetic patients was also observed in the TACTICS-TIMI (Treat Angina with Aggrastat and Determine the Cost of Therapy with an Invasive or Conservative Strategy) 18 trial; diabetic patients had a greater absolute reduction in death or MI with the early invasive strategy (ARR: 7.6% [diabetics] vs. 3.5% [total study population]) [32].

Adjunctive medical therapy for patients with diabetes and ACS

Intravenous GPIIb/IIIa receptor inhibitors for NSTE-ACS

Intravenous GPIIb/IIIa inhibitors reduce the frequency of death, MI, and recurrent ischemia when used as a primary therapy for patients presenting with NSTE-ACS (eptifibatide and tirofiban) and when used as an adjunct to PCI (abciximab and eptifibatide) [33,34]. The benefits of GPIIb/IIIa inhibitors for the initial medical treatment of NSTE-ACS are particularly apparent in patients with high-risk clinical features, including ST-segment deviation on the presenting ECG, positive cardiac markers, and diabetes.

In the PRISM-PLUS (Platelet Receptor Inhibition in Ischemic Syndrome Management in Patients Limited by Unstable Signs and Symptoms) trial, Theroux et al. investigated the benefit of tirofiban in addition to standard antithrombotic therapy for the treatment of NSTE-ACS [35]. Of the 1,570 patients enrolled in the study, 362 had diabetes (23%). The rate of the primary endpoint – death, MI, or refractory ischemia at 6 months – was higher in diabetic than nondiabetic patients (36.2% vs. 28.1%, $P = 0.01$). The rate of death or MI in diabetic patients at 6 months was significantly reduced with tirofiban compared with diabetics receiving standard antithrombotic therapy only (19.2% vs. 11.2%, $P = 0.03$), and the relative treatment effect of tirofiban was greater in diabetic compared with nondiabetic patients ($P = 0.007$ for interaction).

Two recent meta-analyses have also demonstrated the benefit of GPIIb/IIIa inhibitors in the treatment of NSTE-ACS [36,37]. Roffi et al. pooled the diabetic populations enrolled in six large-scale NSTE-ACS trials evaluating the use of these agents. Among 6,458 diabetic patients, treatment with GPIIb/IIIa inhibitors was associated with a significant reduction in mortality at 30 days (OR: 0.74, 95% CI: 0.59–0.92, $P = 0.001$) (see **Figure 4**). In contrast, there was no apparent survival benefit with these agents in nondiabetic patients. The interaction between GPIIb/IIIa inhibitor

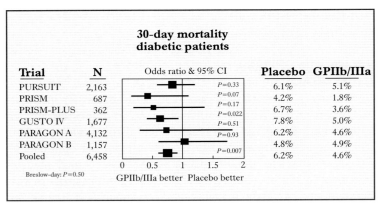

Figure 4. Impact of glycoprotein (GP)IIb/IIIa inhibitors on early mortality in patients with diabetes presenting with non-ST-segment elevation acute coronary syndrome. Adapted with permission from Roffi M, Chew DP, Mukherjee D et al. Platelet glycoprotein IIb/IIIa inhibitors reduce mortality in diabetic patients with non-ST-segment-elevation acute coronary syndromes. *Circulation* 2001;104:2767–71.

use and diabetes was statistically significant ($P = 0.036$). The reduction in 30-day mortality with GPIIb/IIIa inhibitors in diabetic patients was especially pronounced among the 1,279 patients who underwent PCI during the initial hospitalization (OR: 0.30, 95% CI: 0.14–0.69, $P = 0.002$) [36].

Likewise, Boersma et al. pooled individual patient data for all participants in the same six large-scale ACS trials. Patients with diabetes treated with GPIIb/IIIa inhibitors (22% of the population) had a higher risk of 30-day death or MI compared with nondiabetic patients (13.7% vs. 10.6%), and diabetics appeared to derive a greater benefit from the use of these agents [37]. These results suggest an important benefit of GPIIb/IIIa inhibitors in the diabetic population presenting with NSTE-ACS, especially in the setting of early angiography and PCI.

Oral antiplatelet therapy

Given the important structural and functional abnormalities in platelets of diabetics, it is not surprising that these patients derive substantial benefit from aspirin therapy for the treatment of coronary disease. In the Anti-Platelet Trialists' Collaboration Group study, aspirin lowered the combined risk of vascular death, MI, and stroke by 19% ($P < 0.01$) in diabetic patients; an estimated 38 vascular events were prevented per 1,000 patients treated [38]. Treatment with thienopyridine derivatives – ticlopidine or clopidogrel (alone or in combination with aspirin) – may provide additional benefit in reducing ischemic events in diabetics. In the CAPRIE (Clopidogrel versus Aspirin in Patients at Risk for Ischemic Events) trial, the absolute benefit of clopidogrel over aspirin was greater in diabetic patients (21% of the total trial population) compared to nondiabetic patients (ARR: 2.1% vs. 0.5%) [39].

The CURE (Clopidogrel in Unstable Angina to Prevent Recurrent Events) trial randomized 12,562 patients within 24 hours of an ACS to combined treatment with clopidogrel and aspirin versus placebo and aspirin for 3–12 months [40]. Patients with diabetes (23% of the total study population) receiving combined clopidogrel and aspirin treatment had higher rates of cardiovascular death, nonfatal MI, and stroke than nondiabetic patients (14.2% vs. 7.9%). However, absolute and relative reductions in the rate of the composite endpoint were similar in patients with and without diabetes receiving combination antiplatelet therapy (ARR: 2.5% vs. 2.0%). These results suggest that combined antiplatelet therapy with aspirin and clopidogrel may be the preferred treatment for eligible patients with diabetes presenting with ACS.

Antithrombin therapy

Unfractionated heparin

Antithrombin therapy with unfractionated heparin (UFH) is commonly used in patients presenting with STEMI. Six trials have compared combined treatment with aspirin and UFH to treatment with aspirin alone in over 68,000 patients (over 90% of whom received concomitant fibrinolytic therapy). The addition of heparin to the treatment regimen was associated with a small reduction in in-hospital mortality compared with aspirin therapy alone (approximately five fewer deaths per 1,000 patients treated). This beneficial effect was tempered by a small increase in the rate of major bleeding events (approximately two per 1,000 patients treated) [41].

Among patients presenting with NSTE-ACS, there is modest clinical trial evidence to support the combined use of UFH and aspirin. Individual trials have been too small to provide unequivocal evidence, though a meta-analysis aggregating data from six trials showed a trend towards a reduced rate of death or MI with aspirin plus UFH compared with aspirin alone [42]. Unfortunately, the use of UFH treatment for STEMI and NSTE-ACS has not been specifically studied in patients with diabetes.

Low-molecular weight heparin

Several large clinical trials have studied low-molecular weight heparin (LMWH) versus UFH in the setting of NSTE-ACS [43,44]. ESSENCE (Efficacy and Safety of Subcutaneous Enoxaparin in Non-Q-wave Coronary Events Study) randomly assigned 3,171 patients with NSTE-ACS to treatment with LMWH (enoxaparin) or UFH. Overall, the rates of death, MI, or recurrent angina at 14 days and 30 days were significantly lower in patients receiving enoxaparin (ARR: 3.2%, $P = 0.019$; ARR: 3.5%, $P = 0.016$, respectively). The treatment effect of enoxaparin among diabetic patients (22% of the total population) was consistent with that observed in the total patient cohort [43].

The TIMI (Thrombolysis in Myocardial Infarction)-IIB trial demonstrated similar results with enoxaparin compared with UFH [44]. Despite the apparent efficacy of LMWH, difficulties with monitoring the level of anticoagulation during PCI have limited the use of LMWH in patients with NSTE-ACS treated with an early invasive management strategy.

Direct thrombin inhibitors

Newer direct antithrombin agents act against both free and clot-bound thrombin, and lack most of the detrimental qualities of heparin. Several direct thrombin inhibitors – lepirudin, hirudin, and bivalirudin – have been evaluated in large-scale trials of patients presenting with both STEMI and NSTE-ACS. The GUSTO-IIb investigators randomized 12,142 patients presenting with NSTE-ACS or STEMI to 72 hours of therapy with either UFH or hirudin [45]. The 30-day rate of death or MI (the primary endpoint) was 8.9% for those receiving hirudin and 9.8% for those receiving heparin (OR: 0.89, 95% CI: 0.79–1.00, $P = 0.06$). The event rates for patients with diabetes were not reported, but the authors did not indicate the presence of an unfavorable interaction between hirudin treatment and diabetic status.

The OASIS (Organization to Assess Strategies for Ischemic Syndromes)-2 investigators randomized 10,141 patients with NSTE-ACS to 72-hour UFH or hirudin. The rate of the primary endpoint – cardiovascular death or MI at 7 days – was not significantly different in the two treatment arms (4.2% [UFH] vs. 3.6% [hirudin], OR: 0.84, 95% CI: 0.69–1.02, $P = 0.078$). In a subgroup analysis of diabetics, there was no evidence of heterogeneity in the relative benefit of hirudin among diabetic patients [46].

Finally, the HERO (Hirulog and Early Reperfusion or Occlusion)-2 investigators studied the effect of bivalirudin versus UFH in the setting of STEMI [47]. Over 17,000 patients were randomly assigned to a 48-hour infusion of bivalirudin or UFH, as well as standard-dose SK. The primary endpoint (30-day mortality) occurred in 10.8% of those receiving bivalirudin and 10.9% of those receiving heparin (ARR: 0.1%, $P = 0.85$). The 30-day mortality rate was substantially greater among diabetic patients receiving bivalirudin versus similarly treated nondiabetic patients (14.9% vs. 9.8%). The use of bivalirudin was associated with a greater ARR of death in diabetic patients than in nondiabetic patients (2.7% vs. 0%) [47].

As more evidence of the safety and efficacy of LMWH in the setting of early angiography and PCI emerges, it is likely that these agents will become the preferred antithrombin treatment for diabetic patients who present with ACS, given the advantages outlined above. The direct thrombin inhibitors have been shown to have only modest benefit beyond UFH in the setting of STEMI and NSTE-ACS, and are likely to remain the anticoagulant of choice only in the setting of heparin-induced thrombocytopenia, or when UFH or LMWH are contraindicated.

Beta-adrenergic antagonists

Physicians often have reservations regarding the use of beta-blockers in diabetic patients because of the perceived risk of masking hypoglycemia and reducing insulin production [3]. However, most studies show equal or greater reductions in mortality and reinfarction with beta-blockers in diabetic compared with nondiabetic patients [48,49]. Malmberg et al. conducted a retrospective review of diabetic patients participating in two trials – the Göteborg Metoprolol and MIAMI (Metoprolol in Acute Myocardial Infarction) trials – where patients with an acute MI were randomized to treatment with metoprolol or placebo [50]. Among the 120 diabetic patients (9% of the total population) in the Göteborg trial, mortality at 3 months was reduced from 17.9% to 7.5% with metoprolol treatment ($P = 0.16$). Among the 413 patients with diabetes in the MIAMI trial, mortality was decreased from 11.3% to 5.7% with metoprolol treatment ($P = 0.06$). In both of these trials, the magnitude of benefit with beta-blockers was substantially greater in diabetics than in nondiabetics.

An analysis for the National Cooperative Cardiovascular Project (CCP) Database provided additional insights into the utilization and benefits of beta-blockers in diabetic patients after MI [51]. Almost 26% of 45,308 Medicare beneficiaries presenting with acute MI without contraindications to beta-blocker therapy were diabetics; however, only 50% of these diabetic patients were prescribed beta-blockers on discharge after MI. After adjusting for demographic and clinical factors, diabetic patients were less likely to receive beta-blockers at discharge than nondiabetic patients (OR: 0.88, 95% CI: 0.82–0.96). The use of beta-blockers was not associated with increased readmission rates for diabetic complications among patients with or without diabetes.

An analysis of patients in the CCP by Gottlieb et al. also demonstrated a significant reduction in mortality in diabetic patients receiving beta-blockers [52]. Thus, the commonly held belief that beta-blockers will increase the rate of diabetic complications and lead to the deterioration of glycemic control has not been demonstrated in clinical studies, and should not preclude the use of these agents in diabetic patients.

ACE inhibitors

Multiple large, randomized clinical trials, collectively enrolling over 100,000 patients, have unequivocally demonstrated improved survival in patients when angiotensin-converting enzyme (ACE)-inhibitor therapy is initiated during or after an acute MI [53]. In a heterogenous, relatively unselected population of patients, mortality and morbidity were reduced when ACE inhibitors were given during the early stages of an MI (within the first 24–36 hours) [54–56]. Mortality and morbidity were also reduced in patients with symptoms or signs of left ventricular dysfunction after an acute MI when ACE-inhibitor therapy was initiated later – after 3–16 days [57–59].

The ACE Inhibitor Myocardial Infarction Collaborative Group recently published a systematic overview of all randomized trials in which ACE-inhibitor treatment was started in the early phase of acute MI and continued for 4–6 weeks [53]. In this large dataset of over 98,000 patients, 30-day mortality was 7.1% in patients treated with ACE inhibitors compared with 7.6% in patients treated with placebo; this corresponds to a 7% relative reduction in mortality ($P < 0.004$), or five deaths prevented per 1,000 patients treated. Among the 5,014 (5.1%) patients with diabetes in this study, the absolute benefits of ACE-inhibitor treatment were greater than in nondiabetics (17.3 lives saved per 1,000 diabetics treated versus 3.2 lives saved per 1,000 nondiabetics treated).

These results indicate that diabetic patients who suffer an acute MI should receive ACE-inhibitor therapy early in the course of their presentation. The use of ACE inhibitors in diabetic patients with NSTE-ACS has not been specifically studied, but a beneficial effect is likely. Diabetics with NSTE-ACS should routinely be treated with ACE-inhibitors, given the established benefit of this therapy in patients with risk factors for, or clinical manifestations of, vascular disease [60].

In MICRO-HOPE (Microalbuminuria, Cardiovascular and Renal Outcomes Substudy of the Heart Outcomes Prevention Efficacy), investigators set out to determine if the ACE inhibitor – ramipril – reduced the risk of cardiovascular and renal disease in the 3,577 diabetic patients participating in the overall HOPE trial [60]. Patients with diabetes included in this study had either a previous cardiovascular event or one other cardiovascular risk factor. In diabetic patients, ramipril was shown to reduce the rate of: the composite endpoint of MI, stroke, or death by 25%; MI by 22%; stroke by 33%; and total mortality by 24% (see **Figure 5**). Ramipril also reduced the rate of overt nephropathy by 24% ($P = 0.027$) [60]. These results confirm that diabetic patients with coronary disease derive substantial benefit from ACE inhibitors, in both the setting of an ACS and established vascular disease.

Lipid-lowering therapy

The benefit of statin treatment for secondary prevention of cardiovascular disease in patients with established coronary disease – both with and without diabetes – has been clearly demonstrated [61]. However, patients who have experienced an ACS in the 3–4 months prior to study enrollment have commonly been excluded from statin studies of patients with existing vascular disease. Given that the highest risk of death and recurrent ischemic events is early after presentation with an ACS, several groups have investigated if early initiation of statin therapy (prior to hospital discharge) could improve outcomes and shorten the time it takes to benefit from treatment with these agents.

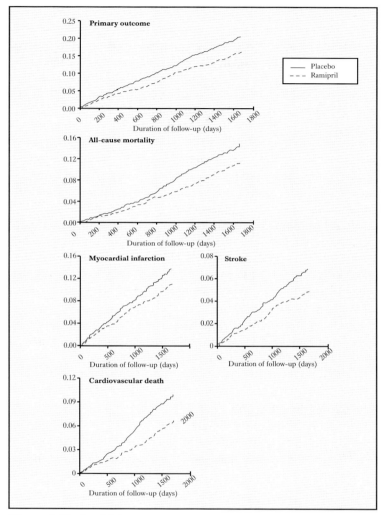

Figure 5. Kaplan–Meier outcome curves from the HOPE trial of diabetic patients. The primary outcome was myocardial infarction, stroke, or cardiovascular death. Adapted with permission from the Heart Outcomes Prevention Evaluation Study Investigators. Effects of ramipril on cardiovascular and microvascular outcomes in people with diabetes mellitus: results of the HOPE study and MICRO-HOPE substudy. *Lancet* 2000;55:253–9.

The MIRACL (Myocardial Ischemia Reduction with Aggressive Lowering) study investigators randomized over 3,000 patients with NSTE-ACS to early treatment, initiated 24–96 hours after hospital admission, with atorvastatin (80 mg/day) or placebo. The rate of the composite primary endpoint – death, nonfatal MI, cardiac arrest, or recurrent ischemia requiring hospitalization – was 14.8% in the atorvastatin-treated group compared with 17.4% in the placebo group (RR: 0.84, 95% CI: 0.70–1.00, $P = 0.48$). This difference in event rates was entirely due to lower rates of recurrent ischemia among those receiving atorvastatin. Though the event rates among the 23% of patients who had diabetes were not reported, there was no significant interaction between treatment assignment and the presence of diabetes, i.e., the presence of diabetes did not affect the relationship between atorvastatin use and the clinical outcome measured [62]. A reduction in the rate of adverse cardiac events was also observed in diabetic patients (12% of the study population) participating in LIPS (the Lescol Intervention Prevention Study), which randomized 1,600 patients after PCI to fluvastatin (80 mg/day) or placebo [63].

The results of MIRACL and LIPS suggest that early initiation of statin therapy after presentation with ACS may reduce the rate of recurrent ischemia requiring hospitalization. Diabetic patients participating in these trials appeared to derive a similar benefit as the overall trial population. The administration of statins prior to discharge in diabetic patients (and all patients) presenting with an ACS may serve to improve the likelihood that these agents will be used in the long term, where their benefits are well established.

Conclusion

CAD is the leading cause of morbidity and mortality among patients with diabetes. In diabetics who present with ACS, the risks of adverse outcomes are much greater than those observed in nondiabetics [64]. Therefore, healthcare providers should remain vigilant when evaluating diabetic patients who seek medical care so that atypical symptoms of myocardial ischemia are not overlooked.

The aggregate clinical trial data to date suggest that diabetics derive a particularly strong benefit from proven therapies, and all attempts should be made to utilize these agents in appropriate patients.

References

1. Garcia MJ, McNamara PM, Gordon T et al. Morbidity and mortality in diabetics in the Framingham population. Sixteen year follow-up study. *Diabetes* 1974;23:105–11.
2. Aronson D, Rayfield EJ, Chesebro JH. Mechanisms determining course and outcome of diabetic patients who have had acute myocardial infarction. *Ann Intern Med* 1997;126:296–306.
3. Beckman JA, Creager MA, Libby P. Diabetes and atherosclerosis: epidemiology, pathophysiology, and management. *JAMA* 2002;287:2570–81.
4. Tschoepe D, Roesen P, Kaufmann L et al. Evidence for abnormal platelet glycoprotein expression in diabetes mellitus. *Eur J Clin Invest* 1990;20:166–70.
5. Aronson D, Bloomgarden Z, Rayfield EJ. Potential mechanisms promoting restenosis in diabetic patients. *J Am Coll Cardiol* 1996;27:528–35.
6. Marchant B, Umachandran V, Stevenson R et al. Silent myocardial ischemia: role of subclinical neuropathy in patients with and without diabetes. *J Am Coll Cardiol* 1993;22:1433–7.
7. Mak KH, Moliterno DJ, Granger CB et al. Influence of diabetes mellitus on clinical outcome in the thrombolytic era of acute myocardial infarction. GUSTO-I Investigators. Global Utilization of Streptokinase and Tissue Plasminogen Activator for Occluded Coronary Arteries. *J Am Coll Cardiol* 1997;30:171–9.
8. The Fibrinolytic Therapy Trialists' (FTT) Collaborative Group. Indications for fibrinolytic therapy in suspected acute myocardial infarction: collaborative overview of early mortality and major morbidity results from all randomised trials of more than 1,000 patients [published correction appears in *Lancet* 1994;343:742]. *Lancet* 1994;343:311–22.
9. Brodie BR, Stuckey TD, Wall TC et al. Importance of time to reperfusion for 30-day and late survival and recovery of left ventricular function after primary angioplasty for acute myocardial infarction. *J Am Coll Cardiol* 1998;32:1312–9.
10. Dracup K, Alonzo AA, Atkins JM et al. The physician's role in minimizing prehospital delay in patients at high risk for acute myocardial infarction: recommendations from the National Heart Attack Alert Program. Working group on educational strategies to prevent prehospital delay in patients at high risk for acute myocardial infarction. *Ann Intern Med* 1997;126:645–51.
11. Kondo T, Kubota I, Tachibana H et al. Glibenclamide attenuates peaked T wave in early phase of myocardial ischemia. *Cardiovasc Res* 1996;31:683–7.
12. Kubota I, Yamaki M, Shibata T et al. Role of ATP-sensitive K$^+$ channel on ECG ST segment elevation during a bout of myocardial ischemia. A study on epicardial mapping in dogs. *Circulation* 1993;88:1845–51.
13. Granger CB, Califf RM, Young S et al. Outcome of patients with diabetes mellitus and acute myocardial infarction treated with thrombolytic agents. The Thrombolysis and Angioplasty in Myocardial Infarction (TAMI) Study Group. *J Am Coll Cardiol* 1999;21:920–5.
14. The GUSTO-III Investigators. A comparison of reteplase with alteplase for acute myocardial infarction. The Global Use of Strategies to Open Occluded Coronary Arteries (GUSTO III) Investigators. *N Engl J Med* 1997;337:1118–23.

15. ASSENT-2 Investigators. Single-bolus tenecteplase compared with front-loaded alteplase in acute myocardial infarction: the ASSENT-2 double-blind randomised trial. *Lancet* 1999;354:716–22.

16. Topol EJ. Reperfusion therapy for acute myocardial infarction with fibrinolytic therapy or combination reduced fibrinolytic therapy and platelet glycoprotein IIb/IIIa inhibition: the GUSTO V randomised trial. *Lancet* 2001;357:1905–14.

17. Pfeffer MA, Moye LA, Braunwald E et al. Selection bias in the use of thrombolytic therapy in acute myocardial infarction. The SAVE Investigators. *JAMA* 1991;266:528–32.

18. Barron HV, Bowlby LJ, Breen T et al. Use of reperfusion therapy for acute myocardial infarction in the United States: data from the National Registry of Myocardial Infarction 2. *Circulation* 1998;97:1150–6.

19. Danchin N, Vaur L, Genes N et al. Treatment of acute myocardial infarction by primary coronary angioplasty or intravenous thrombolysis in the "real world": one-year results from a nationwide French survey. *Circulation* 1999;99:2639–44.

20. Menown I, Patterson R, McMechan S et al. Use of thrombolytic therapy in females, diabetics and the elderly: trial selection – bias or a real problem? *J Am Coll Cardiol* 1999;33:325A.

21. Mahaffey KW, Granger CB, Toth CA et al. Diabetic retinopathy should not be a contraindication to thrombolytic therapy for acute myocardial infarction: review of ocular hemorrhage incidence and location in the GUSTO-I trial. Global Utilization of Streptokinase and t-PA for Occluded Coronary Arteries. *J Am Coll Cardiol* 1997;30:1606–10.

22. Weaver WD, Simes RJ, Betriu A et al. Comparison of primary coronary angioplasty and intravenous thrombolytic therapy for acute myocardial infarction: a quantitative review [published correction appears in *JAMA* 1998;279:1876]. *JAMA* 1997;278:2093–8.

23. Hasdai D, Granger CB, Srivatsa SS et al. Diabetes mellitus and outcome after primary coronary angioplasty for acute myocardial infarction: lessons from the GUSTO-IIb Angioplasty Substudy. Global Use of Strategies to Open Occluded Arteries in Acute Coronary Syndromes [published correction appears in *J Am Coll Cardiol* 2000;36:659]. *J Am Coll Cardiol* 2000;35:1502–12.

24. Brener SJ, Ellis SG, Sapp SK et al. Predictors of death and reinfarction at 30 days after primary angioplasty: the GUSTO IIb and RAPPORT trials. *Am Heart J* 2000;139: 476–81.

25. Stone GW, Grines CL, Browne KF et al. Predictors of in-hospital and 6-month outcome after acute myocardial infarction in the reperfusion era: the Primary Angioplasty in Myocardial Infarction (PAMI) trail. *J Am Coll Cardiol* 1995;25:370–7.

26. Thomas K, Ottervanger JP, de Boer MJ et al. Primary angioplasty compared with thrombolysis in acute myocardial infarction in diabetic patients. *Diabetes Care* 1999;22:647–9.

27. Van De Werf F, Baim DS. Reperfusion for ST-segment elevation myocardial infarction: an overview of current treatment options. *Circulation* 2002;105:2813–6.

38. Stone GW, Grines CL, Cox DA et al. Comparison of angioplasty with stenting, with or without abciximab, in acute myocardial infarction. *N Engl J Med* 2002; 346:957–66.

29. Montalescot G, Barragan P, Wittenberg O et al. Platelet glycoprotein IIb/IIIa inhibition with coronary stenting for acute myocardial infarction. *N Engl J Med* 2001;344:1895–903.

30. Silva JA, Nunez E, White CJ et al. Predictors of stent thrombosis after primary stenting for acute myocardial infarction. *Catheter Cardiovasc Interv* 1999;47:415–22.

31. Invasive compared with non-invasive treatment in unstable coronary-artery disease: FRISC II prospective randomised multicentre study. Fragmin and Fast Revascularisation during Instability in Coronary Artery Disease Investigators. *Lancet* 1999;354:708–15.

32. Cannon CP, Weintraub WS, Demopoulos LA et al. Comparison of early invasive and conservative strategies in patients with unstable coronary syndromes treated with the glycoprotein IIb/IIIa inhibitor tirofiban. *N Engl J Med* 2001;344:1879–87.

33. Kong DF, Califf RM. Glycoprotein IIb/IIIa receptor antagonists in non-ST elevation acute coronary syndromes and percutaneous revascularisation: a review of trial reports. *Drugs* 1999;58:609–20.

34. Kong DF, Califf RM, Miller DP et al. Clinical outcomes of therapeutic agents that block the platelet glycoprotein IIb/IIIa integrin in ischemic heart disease. *Circulation* 1998;98:2829–35.

35. Theroux P, Alexander J Jr, Pharand C et al. Glycoprotein IIb/IIIa receptor blockade improves outcomes in diabetic patients presenting with unstable angina/non-ST-elevation myocardial infarction: results from the Platelet Receptor Inhibition in Ischemic Syndrome Management in Patients Limited by Unstable Signs and Symptoms (PRISM-PLUS) study. *Circulation* 2000;102:2466–72.

36. Boersma E, Harrington RA, Moliterno DJ et al. Platelet glycoprotein IIb/IIIa inhibitors in acute coronary syndromes: a meta-analysis of all major randomised clinical trials [published correction appears in *Lancet* 2002;359:2120]. *Lancet* 2002;359:189–98.

37. Roffi M, Chew DP, Mukherjee D et al. Platelet glycoprotein IIb/IIIa inhibitors reduce mortality in diabetic patients with non-ST-segment-elevation acute coronary syndromes. *Circulation* 2001;104:2767–71.

38. Collaborative overview of randomised trials of antiplatelet therapy – I: Prevention of death, myocardial infarction, and stroke by prolonged antiplatelet therapy in various categories of patients. Anti-platelet Trialists' Collaboration [published correction appears in *BMJ* 1994;308:1540]. *BMJ* 1994;308:81–106.

39. A randomised, blinded, trial of clopidogrel versus aspirin in patients at risk of ischaemic events (CAPRIE). CAPRIE Steering Committee. *Lancet* 1996;348:1329–39.

40. Yusuf S, Zhao F, Mehta SR et al. Effects of clopidogrel in addition to aspirin in patients with acute coronary syndromes without ST-segment elevation [published correction appears in *N Engl J Med* 2001;345:1716, *N Engl J Med* 2001;345:1506]. *N Engl J Med* 2001;345:494–502.

41. Collins R, MacMahon S, Flather M et al. Clinical effects of anticoagulant therapy in suspected acute myocardial infarction: systematic overview of randomised trials. *BMJ.* 1996;313:652–9.

42. Oler A, Whooley MA, Oler J et al. Adding heparin to aspirin reduces the incidence of myocardial infarction and death in patients with unstable angina. A meta-analysis. *JAMA* 1996;276:811–5.

43. Cohen M, Demers C, Gurfinkel EP et al. A comparison of low-molecular-weight heparin with unfractionated heparin for unstable coronary artery disease. Efficacy and Safety of Subcutaneous Enoxaparin in Non-Q-Wave Coronary Events Study Group. *N Engl J Med* 1997;337:447–52.

44. Antman EM, McCabe CH, Gurfinkel EP et al. Enoxaparin prevents death and cardiac ischemic events in unstable angina/non-Q-wave myocardial infarction. Results of the thrombolysis in myocardial infarction (TIMI) 11B trial. *Circulation* 1999;100:1593–601.

45. Metz BK, White HD, Granger CB et al. Randomized comparison of direct thrombin inhibition versus heparin in conjunction with fibrinolytic therapy for acute myocardial infarction: results from the GUSTO-IIb Trial. Global Use of Strategies to Open Occluded Coronary Arteries in Acute Coronary Syndromes (GUSTO-IIb) Investigators. *J Am Coll Cardiol* 1998;31:1493–8.

46. Effects of recombinant hirudin (lepirudin) compared with heparin on death, myocardial infarction, refractory angina, and revascularisation procedures in patients with acute myocardial ischaemia without ST elevation: a randomised trial. Organisation to Assess Strategies for Ischemic Syndromes (OASIS-2) Investigators. *Lancet* 1999;353:429–38.

47. White H. Thrombin-specific anticoagulation with bivalirudin versus heparin in patients receiving fibrinolytic therapy for acute myocardial infarction: the HERO-2 randomised trial. *Lancet* 2001;358:1855–63.

48. Gullestad L, Kjekshus J. [Myocardial disease in diabetes mellitus] [Norwegian]. *Tidsskr Nor Laegeforen* 1992;112:1016–9.

49. Kendall MJ, Lynch KP, Hjalmarson A et al. Beta-blockers and sudden cardiac death. *Ann Intern Med* 1995;123:358–67.

50. Malmberg K, Herlitz J, Hjalmarson A et al. Effects of metoprolol on mortality and late infarction in diabetics with suspected acute myocardial infarction. Retrospective data from two large studies. *Eur Heart J* 1989;10:423–8.

51. Chen J, Marciniak TA, Radford MJ et al. Beta-blocker therapy for secondary prevention of myocardial infarction in elderly diabetic patients. Results from the National Cooperative Cardiovascular Project. *J Am Coll Cardiol* 1999;34:1388–94.

52. Gottlieb SS, McCarter RJ, Vogel RA. Effect of beta-blockade on mortality among high-risk and low-risk patients after myocardial infarction. *N Engl J Med* 1998;339:489–97.

53. Indications for ACE inhibitors in the early treatment of acute myocardial infarction: systematic overview of individual data from 100,000 patients in randomized trials. ACE Inhibitor Myocardial Infarction Collaborative Group. *Circulation* 1998;97:2202–12.

54. Swedberg K, Held P, Kjekshus J et al. Effects of the early administration of enalapril on mortality in patients with acute myocardial infarction. Results of the Cooperative New Scandinavian Enalapril Survival Study II (CONSENSUS II). *N Engl J Med* 1992;327:678–84.

55. GISSI-3: effects of lisinopril and transdermal glyceryl trinitrate singly and together on 6-week mortality and ventricular function after acute myocardial infarction. Gruppo Italiano per lo Studio della Sopravvivenza nell'infarto Miocardico. *Lancet* 1994;343:1115–22.

56. ISIS-4: a randomised factorial trial assessing early oral captopril, oral mononitrate, and intravenous magnesium sulphate in 58,050 patients with suspected acute myocardial infarction. ISIS-4 (Fourth International Study of Infarct Survival) Collaborative Group. *Lancet* 1995;345:669–85.

57. Pfeffer MA, Braunwald E, Moye LA et al. Effect of captopril on mortality and morbidity in patients with left ventricular dysfunction after myocardial infarction. Results of the survival and ventricular enlargement trial. The SAVE Investigators. *N Engl J Med* 1992;327:669–77.

58. Effect of ramipril on mortality and morbidity of survivors of acute myocardial infarction with clinical evidence of heart failure. The Acute Infarction Ramipril Efficacy (AIRE) Study Investigators. *Lancet* 1993;342:821–8.

59. Gustafsson I, Torp-Pedersen C, Kober L et al. Effect of the angiotensin-converting enzyme inhibitor trandolapril on mortality and morbidity in diabetic patients with left ventricular dysfunction after acute myocardial infarction. Trace Study Group. *J Am Coll Cardiol* 1999;34:83–9.

60. Effects of ramipril on cardiovascular and microvascular outcomes in people with diabetes mellitus: results of the HOPE study and MICRO-HOPE substudy. Heart Outcomes Prevention Evaluation Study Investigators [published correction appears in *Lancet* 2000;356:860]. *Lancet* 2000;355:253–9.

61. Grundy SM, Garber A, Goldberg R et al. Prevention Conference VI: Diabetes and Cardiovascular Disease: Writing Group IV: lifestyle and medical management of risk factors. *Circulation* 2002;105:e153–8.

62. Schwartz GG, Olsson AG, Ezekowitz MD et al. Effects of atorvastatin on early recurrent ischemic events in acute coronary syndromes: the MIRACL study: a randomized controlled trial. *JAMA* 2001;285:1711–8.

63. Serruys PW, Feyter P, Macaya C et al. Fluvastatin for prevention of cardiac events following successful first percutaneous coronary intervention: a randomized controlled trial. *JAMA* 2002;287:3215–22.

64. Mak KH, Topol EJ. Emerging concepts in the management of acute myocardial infarction in patients with diabetes mellitus. *J Am Coll Cardiol* 2000;35:563–8.

7

Coronary revascularization in the diabetic patient

Joel P Reginelli & Deepak L Bhatt

Introduction

Although patients with diabetes present a number of challenges to the treating physician, one of the most important therapeutic decisions lies in determining the appropriate timing and modality of coronary revascularization. Given the alarming rise in both the incidence and prevalence of diabetes and insulin-resistance syndrome in the US [1,2] – along with the propensity of these patients to develop diffuse coronary atherosclerotic disease [3] – it is imperative that treating physicians be cognizant of the advantages and disadvantages associated with both surgical and percutaneous revascularization strategies. This is no small order given the wealth of existing – and often conflicting – clinical trial data, the multitude of ongoing studies, and the staggering rate of technological advances that inevitably outpace the results of clinical trials.

The goal of this chapter is to briefly discuss the deleterious effects of diabetic pathophysiology on outcomes following both percutaneous coronary intervention (PCI) and coronary artery bypass grafting (CABG), to summarize the existing clinical trial data, and to discuss ongoing and upcoming trials that may reshape thinking on this controversial topic.

The impact of diabetes on PCI

Since the advent of percutaneous transluminal coronary angioplasty (PTCA) over 2 decades ago, it has been recognized that diabetics are at increased risk for adverse outcomes following percutaneous coronary revascularization (see **Figure 1**) [4,5]. For example, data from an early NHLBI (National Heart, Lung, and Blood Institute) registry demonstrated that – despite similar procedural success rates – diabetics experienced a nearly 2-fold increased risk of both short- and long-term adverse outcomes. The incidence of myocardial infarction (MI), emergent CABG, and in-hospital death was 11% for diabetics compared to 6.7% for nondiabetics (odds ratio [OR]: 1.74, $P < 0.01$), and the 9-year mortality rate was 35.9% for diabetics as opposed to 17.9% for nondiabetics (OR: 2.28, $P < 0.001$) [6].

The development of intracoronary stents represented a quantum leap forward in PCI technology. The use of stents during PCI has been associated with improved outcomes in nearly every patient subgroup, irrespective of the clinical presentation or lesion characteristics. Despite the optimism generated by an early study, which suggested that stenting may equalize PCI outcomes among diabetics and nondiabetics [7], subsequent trials have demonstrated that, although stent use resulted in a relative improvement in outcomes compared to PTCA, diabetics continued to fare worse than their nondiabetic peers [8–10]. It is thought that these discrepant results are due to the unique anatomic and metabolic milieu created by the pathophysiological changes associated with diabetes.

Hyperglycemia is the hallmark of diabetes and has served as a principal treatment target to reduce the incidence of microvascular complications, such as retinopathy, nephropathy, and neuropathy [11]. Although the pathogenic role of hyperglycemia in macrovascular disease is a topic of debate, a clear correlation does exist between hyperglycemia and cardiovascular events [12,13]. Many postulate that hyperglycemia impacts on macrovascular disease – particularly coronary atherosclerotic disease – indirectly through the production of advanced glycation endproducts (AGEs) [14].

AGEs act in a multitude of ways to impair endothelial function, stimulate subendothelial cellular proliferation, and amplify vascular

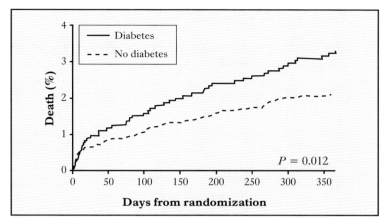

Figure 1. Mortality at 1 year following percutaneous coronary intervention based on diabetic status. Reprinted with permission from Bhatt DL, Marso SP, Lincoff AM et al. Abciximab reduces mortality in diabetics following percutaneous coronary intervention. *J Am Coll Cardiol* 2000;35:922–8.

inflammation [15–17]. These pathogenic mechanisms may underlie the diabetic predilection for aggressive coronary atherosclerotic disease, coronary embolization, impaired coronary collateral formation, decreased coronary flow reserve, and increased rates of restenosis [4,18–22].

These anatomic obstacles to obtaining optimal PCI results are further compounded by the detrimental effects of diabetes on coagulation and platelet function. Diabetes induces a relative hypercoagulable state through the overproduction of procoagulant proteins and underproduction of anticoagulant proteins [23–25]. The diabetic platelet adds to the procoagulant condition due to its large size, increased numbers of platelet glycoprotein (GP)IIb/IIIa receptors, and exaggerated reactivity [26,27]. These alterations in coagulation and platelet function help to explain the high rates of restenosis, and propensity for death due to acute thrombotic events, observed among diabetic patients with cardiovascular disease (CVD) [28].

The impact of diabetes on CABG

The deleterious effects of the proinflammatory and hypercoagulable state associated with diabetes extend to outcomes from CABG. Diabetics undergoing CABG are at substantially increased risk for both short- and long-term adverse events [29–34].

In a study of 1,805 diabetic patients undergoing CABG, Weintraub and associates found that diabetics suffered a higher in-hospital mortality rate than nondiabetics (4.99% vs. 0.36%, $P < 0.0001$) [32]. Thourani and colleagues validated these findings with the observation that diabetics undergoing CABG experienced both an increased rate of in-hospital death (3.9% vs. 1.6%, $P < 0.05$) and perioperative stroke (2.9% vs. 1.4%, $P < 0.05$) [31]. In addition to in-hospital death and stroke, observational studies suggest that diabetics are at higher risk of developing perioperative pulmonary edema, renal insufficiency, and sternal wound infections [30,35].

It has been suggested that these findings are largely attributable to the fact that diabetics undergoing CABG tend to have more diffuse atherosclerotic disease, poorer left ventricular systolic function, and more severe comorbid disease compared to their nondiabetic peers. However, it is generally agreed that these differences in baseline characteristics do not fully explain the disparity of results.

In addition to an increased risk for adverse perioperative events, diabetics also experience inferior long-term outcomes following CABG [30–32,36]. As an example, Thourani and colleagues found that diabetics had a significant reduction in both 5-year and 10-year survival following CABG compared to nondiabetics (78% vs. 88%, $P \leq 0.05$ and 50% vs. 71%, $P \leq 0.05$, respectively) [31]. Several theories have been suggested to explain this survival disadvantage, including: progression of native coronary atherosclerotic disease; silent ischemia leading to left ventricular dysfunction; and the increased prevalence of severe comorbid conditions.

Despite potential shortcomings, CABG has historically been regarded as the revascularization strategy of choice for diabetics with multivessel disease. Although CABG was the only revascularization option until the early 1980s, the arrival of PTCA ushered in a new era of coronary revascularization. Investigators sought to determine whether PTCA was a viable alternative to CABG for patients with symptomatic coronary disease – particularly for diabetics and other high-risk operative candidates.

CABG versus PTCA

Soon after its inception, PTCA became the preferred mode of revascularization for most patients with single-vessel coronary artery disease (CAD). Meanwhile, several trials were designed to determine whether this new modality might provide outcomes equivalent to CABG in patients with multivessel CAD [34,37,38]. As a general rule, these studies demonstrated equivalence of the two strategies with regard to MI, stroke, and death. However, PTCA was consistently associated with markedly increased rates of repeat revascularization. Although these conclusions were based on the study population as a whole, retrospective analyses of the diabetic subsets within these trials have yielded important new insights.

In the CABRI (Coronary Angioplasty versus Bypass Revascularization Investigation) trial, 1,054 patients with multivessel CAD were randomized to either PTCA or CABG. Although mortality at 1 year was similar for both groups (PTCA: 3.9% vs. CABG: 2.7%, $P = 0.297$), recurrent angina and the need for subsequent revascularization was significantly higher among those patients randomized to PTCA [37]. Diabetics represented only 11.9% of the CABRI patient population (n = 125), but there did appear to be a survival benefit at 4 years among those diabetics randomized to CABG rather than PTCA (87.5% vs. 77.4%, respectively) [39].

EAST (the Emory Angioplasty Surgery Trial) randomized 392 patients with multivessel CAD to either PTCA or CABG. The results of EAST mirrored those of CABRI: at 3 years there was no significant difference in mortality between the two treatments (PTCA: 7.1% vs. CABG: 6.2%, $P = 0.73$), but the rates of subsequent angina and revascularization were substantially higher among those patients randomized to PTCA [38]. Only 59 of the patients enrolled in EAST were diabetic, but among this subgroup there was a strong trend toward improved survival at 8 years for those randomized to CABG as opposed to PTCA (75.5% vs. 60.1%, respectively, $P = 0.23$) [40].

The findings of EAST and CABRI were validated in the large-scale BARI (Bypass Angioplasty Revascularization Investigation) trial, which randomized 1,829 patients with multivessel CAD to either PTCA (n = 915) or CABG (n = 914). Although similar rates of in-hospital stroke and death were observed with both treatments, periprocedural MI was more common among those randomized to CABG (4.6% vs. 2.1%, $P < 0.01$) [41]. There was no significant difference in overall survival at 5 years (89.3% vs. 86.3%, $P = 0.19$), but the rate of repeat revascularization was markedly higher among those initially randomized to PTCA (54% vs. 8%, $P < 0.001$). Survival of diabetics was significantly higher among those randomized to CABG rather than PTCA (80.6% vs. 65.5%, respectively, $P = 0.0024$) [42].

A subsequent analysis at 7 years observed a significant survival advantage in the overall study population associated with randomization to CABG (84.4% vs. 80.9%, $P = 0.043$) [43]. It is noteworthy that this survival benefit was driven solely by the outcome of the 353 diabetic patients enrolled in the trial (PTCA: 55.7% vs. CABG: 76.4%, $P = 0.0011$), whereas there was no difference in survival among the 1,476 patients without diabetes (PTCA: 86.8% vs. CABG: 86.4%, $P = 0.72$) [43].

It has been postulated that the long-term survival benefit observed among diabetics randomized to CABG in the BARI trial may be due to a more complete revascularization achieved with CABG. Given the propensity of diabetics for accelerated atherosclerosis and

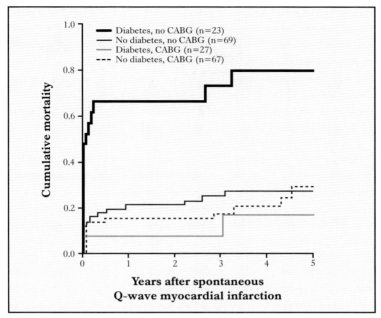

Figure 2. Long-term survival following a Q-wave myocardial infarction in BARI patients stratified by diabetic status and history of coronary artery bypass grafting (CABG). Reprinted with permission from Detre KM, Lombardero MS, Brooks MM et al. The effect of previous coronary-artery bypass surgery on the prognosis of patients with diabetes who have acute myocardial infarction. Bypass Angioplasty Revascularization Investigation Investigators. *N Engl J Med* 2000;342:989–97.

plaque rupture, it follows that complete revascularization may confer additional protection in the setting of future acute coronary events. Data from the BARI trial and registry revealed a substantial survival advantage among diabetics who subsequently suffered a Q-wave MI when randomized to CABG as opposed to PTCA (83% vs. 20%, respectively, $P < 0.001$) (see **Figure 2**) [44]. It is noteworthy that the survival benefit associated with CABG was almost entirely limited to those who had received at least one internal thoracic artery bypass graft.

The importance of placing arterial conduits when performing CABG on diabetic patients was further reinforced in a study by Yamamoto and colleagues, which demonstrated an equivalent long-term survival among diabetics and nondiabetics when an internal thoracic artery conduit was placed [45]. Given the long-term survival benefit conferred by arterial conduits, concerns regarding a potentially increased risk of sternal wound infection should not preclude the use of these grafts in diabetics undergoing CABG [46,47].

The results of the aforementioned trials support the use of CABG for diabetics with multivessel CAD; however, several issues warrant consideration. First, it should be emphasized that concerns have been raised regarding the applicability of these results to "real world" practice. Over 91,000 patients were screened for enrollment in the six major trials that compared CABG to PTCA, of which only 2,943 (5.2%) met criteria for enrollment [48].

Approximately 30% of patients eligible for BARI were ultimately randomized, whereas the remainder elected to choose their mode of revascularization. The BARI registry followed outcomes in over 2,000 of these nonrandomized patients, of whom 339 were diabetic. In contrast to the dramatic improvement in 5-year survival observed among diabetics randomized to CABG (PTCA: 65.5% vs. CABG: 80.6%, $P = 0.0024$), there was no such survival benefit observed among diabetics followed in the registry (PTCA: 85.6% vs. CABG: 85.1%, $P = 0.86$) [49]. Such inconsistent findings raise concerns over the general applicability of the results from the randomized portion of the study.

A second concern over implementing the results of the aforementioned trials is the lightning speed with which technological advances have rendered these data obsolete. Interim advances in surgical techniques, such as off-pump procedures, minimally invasive approaches, and total arterial revascularization have been paralleled by the introduction of intracoronary stents and a rapidly expanding pharmacologic armamentarium for improved outcomes with PCI.

CABG versus contemporary PCI

The field of interventional cardiology was revolutionized by the introduction of intracoronary stents This new technology improved procedural success rates, allowed operators to approach anatomy that was previously deemed too high risk, and resulted in improved long-term outcomes following PCI – namely, decreased restenosis and the need for target vessel revascularization (TVR) [7,50–54]. Since restenosis and TVR represented the major limitations of PTCA in the earlier comparative trials with CABG, investigators undertook several trials to determine if stents might succeed in leveling the playing field between PCI and CABG in patients with multivessel disease.

ARTS (the Arterial Revascularization Therapies Study) randomized 1,205 patients with symptomatic multivessel CAD to either CABG or PCI with stenting. At 1 year, there was no difference in the rate of stroke, MI, or death with the two treatments; however, PCI was associated with a significant increase in the need for TVR (PCI: 21% vs. CABG: 3.8%, $P < 0.001$) [55]. A subgroup analysis of the 208 diabetic patients enrolled in ARTS revealed that event-free survival at 1 year was highest among the diabetics randomized to CABG (CABG: 84.4% vs. PCI: 63.4%, $P < 0.001$) [55,56]. Analogous to observations from the earlier PTCA versus CABG trials, this discrepancy in long-term outcomes was driven almost exclusively by the increased need for TVR among diabetics randomized to PCI.

As with ARTS, patients with multivessel disease in the ERACI (Argentine Randomized Study of Coronary Angioplasty with Stenting versus Coronary Artery Bypass Surgery in Patients with Multiple-Vessel Disease)-II and the SOS (Stent or Surgery) trials were randomized to undergo PCI with stenting or CABG [57,58]. The SOS trial, which randomized 988 patients, observed no significant difference in the rate of death or MI; however, the need for repeat revascularization was substantially higher with PCI (PCI: 21% vs. CABG: 6%, $P < 0.0001$) [57].

Although the ERACI-II trial was smaller than ARTS and SOS (N = 450), it enrolled a higher-risk patient population, as evidenced by the fact that over 90% of the patients presented with unstable angina. The findings of ERACI-II were consistent with both ARTS and SOS in that the need for repeat revascularization was highest with PCI (PCI: 16.8% vs. CABG: 4.8%, $P < 0.002$); however, this trial differed substantially from the others in observing an overall survival advantage with PCI (PCI: 96.9% vs. CABG: 92.5%, $P < 0.017$) [58]. Diabetics constituted 15%–17% of the patient population in each of these two trials, but, as yet, diabetic subgroup analyses have not been published.

The weight of evidence from these trials suggests that contemporary PCI and CABG result in similar rates of procedural success and long-term survival; however, patients undergoing PCI are much more likely to require subsequent revascularization procedures. Although data specific to diabetics with multivessel disease are somewhat sparse, those available from ARTS and the earlier PTCA trials favor CABG as the preferred mode of revascularization. However, several limitations of these data must be kept in mind. Each of these studies randomized only a small percentage of those screened, thus, once again, raising concerns over general applicability to real – world medical practice. Of greatest concern is that none of these trials reflect the tremendous advances in PCI therapy that have occurred over the last few years – namely, the widespread use of intravenous platelet GPIIb/IIIa inhibitors, the effectiveness of vascular brachytherapy for in-stent restenosis, and the stunning results recently obtained with the use of drug-eluting stents.

Glycoprotein IIb/IIIa inhibitors

As platelet activation and aggregation following trauma to the endothelium serves as a catalyst for thrombin generation, the platelet is an attractive target for therapeutics directed at reducing thrombotic complications during PCI. The platelet GPIIb/IIIa inhibitors were developed in an attempt to block the final common pathway of platelet aggregation and activation [59].

Abciximab, the first commercially available GPIIb/IIIa inhibitor, has been shown to improve outcomes across a broad range of patients undergoing PTCA or PCI with stenting [60–62]. The "small-molecule" GPIIb/IIIa inhibitors – eptifibatide and tirofiban – were not effective in improving outcomes during PTCA [63,64]; however, recent coronary stenting trials have demonstrated a clinical benefit with the use of these agents [65,66].

The EPISTENT (Evaluation of Platelet IIb/IIIa Inhibitor for Stenting) trial randomized 2,399 patients to one of the following treatments: stent with abciximab (S + A), stent with placebo (S + P), or PTCA with abciximab (PTCA + A). Combined treatment with stenting and abciximab was associated with a significant reduction in death, MI, or TVR at 6 months, and the magnitude of benefit with this combination appeared to be greatest in the subset of patients with diabetes.

In the diabetic substudy of EPISTENT, the combination of abciximab and stenting had the following effects: an approximate 50% relative reduction in the composite endpoint at 6 months (S + A: 13% vs. S + P: 25.2% vs. PTCA + A: 23.4%, $P < 0.001$ and $P = 0.007$) (see **Figure 3**), a trend toward improved mortality rates at 1 year (S + A: 1.2% vs. S + P: 4.1% vs. PTCA + A: 2.6%, $P = 0.11$), and the potential to eradicate the excess 1-year mortality in diabetics undergoing PCI (diabetic: 1.2% vs. nondiabetic: 1.0%) [67].

A pooled analysis was performed on a total of 6,538 patients enrolled in the three major abciximab PCI trials – EPIC (the Evaluation of c7E3 for the Prevention of Ischemic Complications), EPILOG (the Evaluation of PTCA to Improve Long-term Outcome with Abciximab GPIIb/IIIa Blockade), and EPISTENT. In the subset analysis of 1,462 diabetic PCI patients, the use of abciximab was associated with a significant reduction in 1-year mortality (abciximab: 2.5% vs. placebo: 4.5%, $P = 0.031$) (see **Figure 4**) [5], and perhaps more relevant to this discussion, diabetics undergoing multivessel PCI (n = 173) appeared to derive the greatest mortality benefit (abciximab: 0.9% vs. placebo: 7.7%, $P = 0.018$) [68].

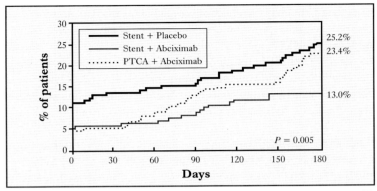

Figure 3. Six-month outcomes among diabetic patients in EPISTENT. Reprinted with permission from Marso SP, Lincoff AM, Ellis SG et al. Optimizing the percutaneous interventional outcomes for patients with diabetes mellitus: results of the EPISTENT (Evaluation of Platelet IIb/IIIa Inhibitor for Stenting) diabetic substudy. *Circulation* 1999;100:2477–84.

It is worth mentioning that GPIIb/IIIa inhibition was used sparingly in the three major trials comparing contemporary PCI to CABG (3.5% in ARTS, 8% in SOS, and 28% in ERACI-II), thus making it difficult to extrapolate the results of those trials to modern day interventional practice.

Device technology

In addition to advances in adjunctive pharmacotherapy, there have recently been two major advances in device technology that may ultimately render data from earlier PCI versus CABG trials obsolete – vascular brachytherapy and drug-eluting stents.

Vascular brachytherapy

The major limitation of multivessel PCI with stent implantation has been the increased need for repeat revascularization procedures due to in-stent restenosis (ISR), especially in diabetic patients whose metabolic milieu appears to promote excessive neointimal formation [69]. The treatment of ISR using conventional PCI methods has proven frustrating due to the high rate of recurrent restenosis;

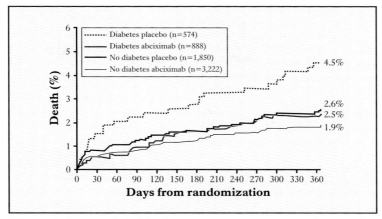

Figure 4. Impact of abciximab on percutaneous coronary intervention outcomes in diabetic patients in EPIC, EPILOG, and EPISTENT. Adapted with permission from Bhatt DL, Marso SP, Lincoff AM et al. Abciximab reduces mortality in diabetics following percutaneous coronary intervention. *J Am Coll Cardiol* 2000;35:922–8.

however, vascular brachytherapy – using both γ and β irradiation – has proven to be an easy and effective therapy [70,71]. Diabetics appear to derive an equal, or greater, benefit from vascular brachytherapy compared to their nondiabetic peers [72]. Even more important than the ability to treat ISR, it appears that prevention is no longer a dream, but rather an imminent reality with the arrival of drug-eluting stents.

Drug-eluting stents

Although several antiproliferative compounds have been tested in a variety of stent delivery systems, to date, the most promising results have come from the sirolimus-coated stent. In the RAVEL (Randomized Study with the Sirolimus-Eluting Velocity Balloon Expandable Stent) trial, the use of sirolimus-coated stents was associated with a remarkable 0% restenosis rate in all 238 patients – including diabetics – compared to a rate of 26% with bare-metal stents ($P < 0.0001$) [73].

The SIRIUS (North American Sirolimus-Eluting Stent) trial randomized a higher-risk patient population with more diffuse and severe CAD. In this trial, the use of sirolimus-coated stents resulted in a significant reduction in the overall rate of restenosis compared to bare-metal stents (8.9% vs. 36.3%, $P < 0.001$) [74]. This finding was consistent across many high-risk subgroups, including diabetics (17.5% vs. 50.5%) [74].

It is important to remember that vascular brachytherapy and drug-eluting stents were not available, and platelet GPIIb/IIIa inhibitors were sparingly used, at the time of the earlier comparison trials between CABG and multivessel PCI; therefore, the impact these modalities may have had on the trial populations as a whole, and diabetics in particular, remains speculative.

Upcoming trials

In the ever-changing field of interventional cardiology, technological advances typically outpace the findings of randomized clinical trials; therefore, establishing a treatment standard of care is a dynamic, and frequently controversial, process. For example, the unprecedented results recently reported with the use of drug-eluting stents will almost certainly call into question any conclusions generated by the earlier CABG versus PCI trials. While it seems likely that a greater percentage of patients with multivessel CAD will now undergo an initial attempt at PCI, it remains unclear whether this will be the best strategy for patients with diabetes.

The upcoming FREEDOM (Future Revascularization Evaluation in Patients with Diabetes Mellitus) trial hopes to shed light on this issue by randomizing diabetics with multivessel CAD to undergo either "state-of-the-art" CABG, including off-pump and complete arterial revascularization procedures, or multivessel PCI using sirolimus-coated stents and adjunctive platelet GPIIb/IIIa inhibitors.

Two additional forthcoming diabetic revascularization trials warrant a mention. In the PPAR (Prevention of Adverse Events following Percutaneous Coronary Revascularization) trial, diabetics undergoing PCI will be randomized to receive placebo or rosiglitazone – a member of the relatively new class of drugs known as thiazolidinediones. The thiazolidinediones are peroxisome proliferator-activated receptor (PPAR)-γ agonists that are rapidly gaining favor in the treatment of diabetes due to their ability to: increase insulin sensitivity; decrease inflammation; and improve endogenous fibrinolysis, glycemic control, and lipoprotein abnormalities [75,78]. It remains to be seen whether these agents might improve outcomes following PCI.

The upcoming BARI 2D (2 Diabetes) trial plans to enroll diabetics with multivessel CAD and stable angina. Patients will be randomized to undergo either revascularization – via CABG or PCI at the discretion of the treating physician – or intensification of medical therapy through either an "insulin-sensitizing" therapy (metformin or a thiazolidinedione) or an "insulin-providing" therapy (sulfonylurea or exogenous insulin).

Additionally, long-term antiplatelet therapy appears to be particularly important in the diabetic. A subgroup analysis from the CAPRIE (Clopidogrel versus Aspirin in Patients at Risk of Ischemic Events) trial demonstrated that diabetics derive particular benefit from treatment with clopidogrel rather than aspirin (see **Figure 5**) [79]. The ongoing CHARISMA (Clopidogrel for High Atherothrombotic Risk and Ischemic Stabilization, Management, and Avoidance) trial will randomize patients with atherosclerotic disease, including those with diabetes, to either combination therapy with clopidogrel and aspirin or monotherapy with aspirin. This trial should help to determine whether dual antiplatelet therapy with aspirin and clopidogrel should become standard of care therapy for patients with diabetes and atherosclerotic disease.

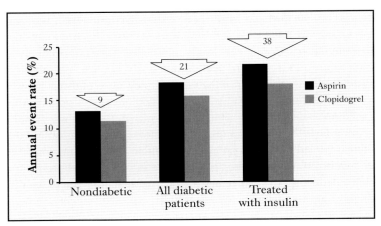

Figure 5. Impact of clopidogrel on vascular events in diabetics enrolled in CAPRIE. The number of events prevented per 1,000 patients per year treated by clopidogrel compared with aspirin. Reprinted with permission from Bhatt D, Marso S, Hirsch A et al. Amplified benefit of clopidogrel versus aspirin in patients with a history of diabetes mellitus. *Am J Cardiol* 2002;90:625–8.

Conclusion

The optimal revascularization strategy for diabetics with multivessel CAD remains a contentious issue. While data from the early PTCA versus CABG trials suggested a long-term benefit with CABG, these trials took place prior to the widespread utilization of intracoronary stents and platelet GPIIb/IIIa inhibitors. To further compound the confusion surrounding this issue, the extraordinary results obtained with drug-eluting stents call into question the relevance of earlier comparison trials.

To assist in making the most appropriate choice for a given patient, it has been suggested that the decision be based more on the coronary anatomy involved, rather than the presence or absence of diabetes. Diabetics with left main trunk stenosis, severe diffuse narrowings involving each of the epicardial vessels, and moderate to severely impaired left ventricular systolic function should be considered for CABG; those whose disease is relatively focal in nature, and does not involve the left main trunk or ostial left anterior descending artery, may be considered for multivessel PCI.

Realistically, once drug-eluting stents are widely available, patients will probably demand PCI over CABG whenever feasible. It is important to remember that, irrespective of whether a diabetic patient is ultimately referred for PCI or CABG, the impact of adjunctive medical therapy is enormous. Given the diabetic proclivity for rapid progression of disease and plaque rupture, strong consideration should be given to initiating drugs of proven benefit in this patient population, namely aspirin, clopidogrel, 3-hydroxy-3-methylglutaryl-coenzyme A (HMG-CoA) reductase inhibitors, beta-blockers, and angiotensin-converting enzyme inhibitors.

References

1. The American Heart Association. 2001 Heart and Stroke Statistical Update. Dallas: American Heart Association, 1999:1–29.
2. Ford ES, Giles WH, Dietz WH. Prevalence of the metabolic syndrome among US adults: findings from the third National Health and Nutrition Examination Survey. *JAMA* 2002;287:356–9.
3. Gu K, Cowie CC, Harris MI. Diabetes and decline in heart disease mortality in US adults. *JAMA* 1999;281:1291–7.
4. Stein B, Weintraub WS, Gebhart SP et al. Influence of diabetes mellitus on early and late outcome after percutaneous transluminal coronary angioplasty. *Circulation* 1995; 91:979–89.
5. Bhatt DL, Marso SP, Lincoff AM et al. Abciximab reduces mortality in diabetics following percutaneous coronary intervention. *J Am Coll Cardiol* 2000;35:922–8.
6. Kip KE, Faxon DP, Detre KM et al. Coronary angioplasty in diabetic patients. The National Heart, Lung, and Blood Institute Percutaneous Transluminal Coronary Angioplasty Registry. *Circulation* 1996;94:1818–25.
7. Van Belle E, Bauters C, Hubert E et al. Restenosis rates in diabetic patients: a comparison of coronary stenting and balloon angioplasty in native coronary vessels. *Circulation* 1997;96:1454–60.
8. Yokoi H, Nosaka H, Kimura T et al. Coronary stenting in diabetic patients: early and follow-up results. *J Am Coll Cardiol* 1997;29:455A.
9. Elezi S, Schulen H, Wehinger A et al. Stent placement in diabetic versus non-diabetic patients. Six-month angiographic follow-up. *J Am Coll Cardiol* 1997:188A.
10. Abizaid A, Kornowski R, Mintz GS et al. The influence of diabetes mellitus on acute and late clinical outcomes following coronary stent implantation. *J Am Coll Cardiol* 1998; 32:584–9.

11. The DCCT Investigators. The effect of intensive treatment of diabetes on the development and progression of long-term complications in insulin-dependent diabetes mellitus. The Diabetes Control and Complications Trial Research Group. *N Engl J Med* 1993;329:977–86.

12. Rodriguez BL, Lau N, Burchfiel CM et al. Glucose intolerance and 23-year risk of coronary heart disease and total mortality: the Honolulu Heart Program. *Diabetes Care* 1999;22:1262–5.

13. Alexander CM, Landsman PB, Teutsch SM. Diabetes mellitus, impaired fasting glucose, atherosclerotic risk factors, and prevalence of coronary heart disease. *Am J Cardiol* 2000;86:897–902.

14. Bierhaus A, Hofmann MA, Ziegler R et al. AGEs and their interaction with AGE-receptors in vascular disease and diabetes mellitus. I. The AGE concept. *Cardiovasc Res* 1998;37:586–600.

15. Schmidt AM, Hori O, Chen JX et al. Advanced glycation endproducts interacting with their endothelial receptor induce expression of vascular cell adhesion molecule-1 (VCAM-1) in cultured human endothelial cells and in mice. A potential mechanism for the accelerated vasculopathy of diabetes. *J Clin Invest* 1995;96:1395–403.

16. Schmidt AM, Stern D. Atherosclerosis and diabetes: the RAGE connection. *Curr Atheroscler Rep* 2000;2:430–6.

17. Yan SD, Schmidt AM, Anderson GM et al. Enhanced cellular oxidant stress by the interaction of advanced glycation end products with their receptors/binding proteins. *J Biol Chem* 1994;269:9889–97.

18. Silva JA, Escobar A, Collins TJ et al. Unstable angina. A comparison of angioscopic findings between diabetic and nondiabetic patients. *Circulation* 1995;92:1731–6.

19. Yokoyama I, Ohtake T, Momomura S et al. Hyperglycemia rather than insulin resistance is related to reduced coronary flow reserve in NIDDM. *Diabetes* 1998;47:119–24.

20. Abaci A, Oguzhan A, Kahraman S et al. Effect of diabetes mellitus on formation of coronary collateral vessels. *Circulation* 1999;99:2239–42.

21. Van Belle E, Abolmaali K, Bauters C et al. Restenosis, late vessel occlusion and left ventricular function six months after balloon angioplasty in diabetic patients. *J Am Coll Cardiol* 1999;34:476–85.

22. Van Belle E, Maillard L, Tio F et al. Accelerated endothelialization by local delivery of recombinant human VEGF reduces in-stent intimal formation. *J Am Coll Cardiol* 1997;29:77A.

23. Ceriello A, Giacomello R, Stel G et al. Hyperglycemia-induced thrombin formation in diabetes. The possible role of oxidative stress. *Diabetes* 1995;44:924–8.

24. Carr ME. Diabetes mellitus: a hypercoagulable state. *J Diabetes Complications* 2001;15:44–54.

25. Nordt TK, Bode C. Impaired endogenous fibrinolysis in diabetes mellitus: mechanisms and therapeutic approaches. *Semin Thromb Hemost* 2000;26:495–501.

26. Knobler H, Savion N, Shenkman B et al. Shear-induced platelet adhesion and aggregation on subendothelium are increased in diabetic patients. *Thromb Res* 1998;90:181–90.

27. Winocour PD. Platelet abnormalities in diabetes mellitus. *Diabetes* 1992;41 (Suppl. 2): 26–31.

28. Tschoepe D, Roesen P. Heart disease in diabetes mellitus: a challenge for early diagnosis and intervention. *Exp Clin Endocrinol Diabetes* 1998;106:16–24.

29. Carson JL, Scholz PM, Chen AY et al. Diabetes mellitus increases short-term mortality and morbidity in patients undergoing coronary artery bypass graft surgery. *J Am Coll Cardiol* 2002;40:418–23.

30. Salomon NW, Page US, Okies JE et al. Diabetes mellitus and coronary artery bypass. Short-term risk and long-term prognosis. *J Thorac Cardiovasc Surg* 1983;85:264–71.

31. Thourani VH, Weintraub WS, Stein B et al. Influence of diabetes mellitus on early and late outcome after coronary artery bypass grafting. *Ann Thorac Surg* 1999;67:1045–52.

32. Weintraub WS, Stein B, Kosinski A et al. Outcome of coronary bypass surgery versus coronary angioplasty in diabetic patients with multivessel coronary artery disease. *J Am Coll Cardiol* 1998;31:10–9.

33. Barsness GW, Peterson ED, Ohman EM et al. Relationship between diabetes mellitus and long-term survival after coronary bypass and angioplasty. *Circulation* 1997;96:2551–6.

34. The BARI Investigators. Influence of diabetes on 5-year mortality and morbidity in a randomized trial comparing CABG and PTCA in patients with multivessel disease: the Bypass Angioplasty Revascularization Investigation (BARI). *Circulation* 1997;96:1761–9.

35. Matsa M, Paz Y, Gurevitch J. Bilateral skeletonized internal thoracic artery grafts in patients with diabetes mellitus. *J Thorac Cardiovasc Surg* 2001;121:668–74.

36. The BARI Investigators. Seven-year outcome in the Bypass Angioplasty Revascularization Investigation (BARI) by treatment and diabetic status. *J Am Coll Cardiol* 2000;35:1122–9.

37. CABRI Trial Participants. First-year results of CABRI (Coronary Angioplasty versus Bypass Revascularization Investigation. *Circulation* 1996;93:847.

38. King SB 3rd, Lembo NJ, Weintraub WS et al. A randomized trial comparing coronary angioplasty with coronary bypass surgery. Emory Angioplasty versus Surgery Trial (EAST). *N Engl J Med* 1994;331:1044–50.

39. Kurbaan AS, Bowker TJ, Ilsley CD et al. Difference in the mortality of the CABRI diabetic and nondiabetic populations and its relation to coronary artery disease and the revascularization mode. *Am J Cardiol* 2001;87:947–50.

40. King SB 3rd, Kosinski AS, Guyton RA et al. Eight-year mortality in the Emory Angioplasty versus Surgery Trial (EAST). *J Am Coll Cardiol* 2000;35:1116–21.

41. The BARI Investigators. Comparison of coronary bypass surgery with angioplasty in patients with multivessel disease. The Bypass Angioplasty Revascularization Investigation (BARI) Investigators. *N Engl J Med* 1996;335:217–25.

42. The BARI Investigators. Five-year clinical and functional outcome comparing bypass surgery and angioplasty in patients with multivessel coronary disease. A multicenter randomized trial. Writing Group for the Bypass Angioplasty Revascularization Investigation (BARI) Investigators. *JAMA* 1997;277:715–21.

43. The BARI Investigators. Seven-year outcome in the Bypass Angioplasty Revascularization Investigation (BARI) by treatment and diabetic status. *J Am Coll Cardiol* 2000;35:1122–9.

44. Detre KM, Lombardero MS, Brooks MM et al. The effect of previous coronary-artery bypass surgery on the prognosis of patients with diabetes who have acute myocardial infarction. Bypass Angioplasty Revascularization Investigation Investigators. *N Engl J Med* 2000;342:989–97.

45. Yamamoto T, Hosoda Y, Takazawa K et al. Is diabetes mellitus a major risk factor in coronary artery bypass grafting? The influence of internal thoracic artery grafting on late survival in diabetic patients. *Jpn J Thorac Cardiovasc Surg* 2000;48:344–52.

46. Wouters R, Wellens F, Vanermen H et al. Sternitis and mediastinitis after coronary artery bypass grafting. Analysis of risk factors. *Tex Heart Inst J* 1994;21:183–8.

47. McDonald WS, Brame M, Sharp C et al. Risk factors for median sternotomy dehiscence in cardiac surgery. *South Med J* 1989;82:1361–4.

48. Sim I, Gupta M, McDonald K et al. A meta-analysis of randomized trials comparing coronary artery bypass grafting with percutaneous transluminal coronary angioplasty in multivessel coronary artery disease. *Am J Cardiol* 1995;76:1025–9.

49. Detre KM, Guo P, Holubkov R et al. Coronary revascularization in diabetic patients: a comparison of the randomized and observational components of the Aypass Angioplasty Revascularization Investigation (BARI). *Circulation* 1999;99:633–40.

50. Fischman DL, Leon MB, Baim DS et al. A randomized comparison of coronary-stent placement and balloon angioplasty in the treatment of coronary artery disease. Stent Restenosis Study Investigators. *N Engl J Med* 1994;331:496–501.

51. Serruys PW, de Jaegere P, Kiemeneij F et al. A comparison of balloon-expandable-stent implantation with balloon angioplasty in patients with coronary artery disease. Benestent Study Group. *N Engl J Med* 1994;331:489–95.

52. Buller CE, Dzavik V, Carere RG et al. Primary stenting versus balloon angioplasty in occluded coronary arteries: the Total Occlusion Study of Canada (TOSCA). *Circulation* 1999;100:236–42.

53. Savage MP, Douglas JS Jr, Fischman DL et al. Stent placement compared with balloon angioplasty for obstructed coronary bypass grafts. Saphenous Vein *De Novo* Trial Investigators. *N Engl J Med* 1997;337:740–7.

54. Versaci F, Gaspardone A, Tomai F et al. A comparison of coronary-artery stenting with angioplasty for isolated stenosis of the proximal left anterior descending coronary artery. *N Engl J Med* 1997;336:817–22.

55. Serruys PW, Unger F, Sousa JE et al. Comparison of coronary-artery bypass surgery and stenting for the treatment of multivessel disease. *N Engl J Med* 2001;344:1117–24.

56. Abizaid A, Costa MA, Centemero M et al. Clinical and economic impact of diabetes mellitus on percutaneous and surgical treatment of multivessel coronary disease patients: insights from the Arterial Revascularization Therapy Study (ARTS) trial. *Circulation* 2001;104:533–8.

57. The SOS Investigators. Coronary artery bypass surgery versus percutaneous coronary intervention with stent implantation in patients with multivessel coronary artery disease (the Stent or Surgery trial): a randomised controlled trial. *Lancet* 2002;360:965–700.

58. Rodriguez A, Bernardi V, Navia J et al. Argentine Randomized Study: Coronary Angioplasty with Stenting versus Coronary Bypass Surgery in patients with Multiple-Vessel Disease (ERACI II): 30-day and one-year follow-up results. ERACI II Investigators. *J Am Coll Cardiol* 2001;37:51–8.

59. Bhatt DL, Topol EJ. Current role of platelet glycoprotein IIb/IIIa inhibitors in acute coronary syndromes. *JAMA* 2000;284:1549–58.

60. The EPIC Investigators. Use of a monoclonal antibody directed against the platelet glycoprotein IIb/IIIa receptor in high-risk coronary angioplasty. *N Engl J Med* 1994;330:956–61.

61. The EPILOG Investigators. Platelet glycoprotein IIb/IIIa receptor blockade and low-dose heparin during percutaneous coronary revascularization. *N Engl J Med* 1997;336:1689–96.

62. The EPISTENT Investigators. Randomised placebo-controlled and balloon-angioplasty-controlled trial to assess safety of coronary stenting with use of platelet glycoprotein-IIb/IIIa blockade. Evaluation of Platelet IIb/IIIa Inhibitor for Stenting. *Lancet* 1998; 352:87–92.

63. The IMPACT-II Investigators. Randomised placebo-controlled trial of effect of eptifibatide on complications of percutaneous coronary intervention. Integrilin to Minimise Platelet Aggregation and Coronary Thrombosis-II. *Lancet* 1997;349:1422–8.

64. The RESTORE Investigators. Effects of platelet glycoprotein IIb/IIIa blockade with tirofiban on adverse cardiac events in patients with unstable angina or acute myocardial infarction undergoing coronary angioplasty. Randomized Efficacy Study of Tirofiban for Outcomes and Restenosis. *Circulation* 1997;96:1445–53.

65. O'Shea JC, Hafley GE, Greenberg S et al. Platelet glycoprotein IIb/IIIa integrin blockade with eptifibatide in coronary stent intervention: the ESPRIT trial: a randomized controlled trial. *JAMA* 2001;285:2468–73.

66. Topol EJ, Moliterno DJ, Herrmann HC et al. Comparison of two platelet glycoprotein IIb/IIIa inhibitors, tirofiban and abciximab, for the prevention of ischemic events with percutaneous coronary revascularization. *N Engl J Med* 2001;344:1888–94.

67. Marso SP, Lincoff AM, Ellis SG et al. Optimizing the percutaneous interventional outcomes for patients with diabetes mellitus: results of the EPISTENT (Evaluation of platelet IIb/IIIa inhibitor for stenting trial) diabetic substudy. *Circulation* 1999;100:2477–84.

68. Bhatt D, Lincoff A, Tcheng J et al. The impact of abciximab on mortality after multivessel PCI: a striking effect in diabetics. *J Am Coll Cardiol* 2000;35:91A.

69. Kornowski R, Mintz GS, Kent KM et al. Increased restenosis in diabetes mellitus after coronary interventions is due to exaggerated intimal hyperplasia. A serial intravascular ultrasound study. *Circulation* 1997;95:1366–9.

70. Waksman R, White R, Chan R et al. Intracoronary gamma-radiation therapy after angioplasty inhibits the recurrence of in-stent restenosis. *Circulation* 2000;101:2165–71.

71. Waksman R, Bhargava B, White L et al. Intracoronary beta-radiation therapy inhibits recurrence of in-stent restenosis. *Circulation* 2000;101:1895–8.

72. Moses JW, Moussa I, Leon MB et al. Effect of catheter-based iridium-192 gamma brachytherapy on the added risk of restenosis from diabetes mellitus after intervention for in-stent restenosis (subanalysis of the GAMMA 1 randomized trial). *Am J Cardiol* 2002;90:243–7.

73. Morice MC, Serruys PW, Sousa JE et al. A randomized comparison of a sirolimus-eluting stent with a standard stent for coronary revascularization. *N Engl J Med* 2002;346: 1773–80.

74. Moses JW. A US Multicenter, Randomized, Double-Blind Study of the Sirolimus-Eluting Stent in *De Novo* Native Coronary Lesions. Washington DC: Transcatheter Cardiovascular Therapeutics, 2002.

75. Marx N, Schonbeck U, Lazar MA et al. Peroxisome proliferator-activated receptor gamma activators inhibit gene expression and migration in human vascular smooth muscle cells. *Circ Res* 1998;83:1097–103.

76. McTernan. Rosiglitazone inhibits the insulin-mediated increase in PAI-1 secretion in human subcutaneous adipocytes. *Diabetes* 2001;50 (Suppl. 2):A275.

77. Aizawa Y, Kawabe J, Hasebe N et al. Pioglitazone enhances cytokine-induced apoptosis in vascular smooth muscle cells and reduces intimal hyperplasia. *Circulation* 2001; 104:455–60.

78. Thomas J, Taylor K. Effects of troglitazone on lipoprotein subclasses in patients who are insulin-resistant. *Diabetes* 2001;50 (Suppl. 2):A455.

79. Bhatt D, Marso S, Hirsch A et al. Amplified benefit of clopidogrel versus aspirin in patients with a history of diabetes mellitus. *Am J Cardiol* 2002;90:625–8.

Abbreviations

ABCD	Appropriate Blood Pressure Control in Diabetics
ACE	angiotensin-converting enzyme
ACS	acute coronary syndrome
ADA	American Diabetes Association
ADMIRAL	Abciximab before Direct Angioplasty and Stenting in Myocardial Infarction Regarding Acute and Long-term Follow-up
ADP	adenosine diphosphate
AGE	advanced glycation endproduct
AHA	American Heart Association
ALLHAT	Antihypertensive and Lipid-lowering Treatment to Prevent Heart Attack Trial
APOB	apolipoprotein B
ARB	angiotensin receptor blocker
ARIC	Atherosclerosis Risk in Communities
ARR	absolute risk reduction
ARTS	Arterial Revascularization Therapies Study
AT_1	angiotensin II tissue receptor subtype I
ATLAS	Assessment of Treatment with Lisinopril and Survival
BARI	Bypass Angioplasty Revascularization Investigation
BP	blood pressure

BUPA	British United Provident Association
CABG	coronary artery bypass grafting
CABRI	Coronary Angioplasty versus Bypass Revascularization Investigation
CAD	coronary artery disease
CADILLAC	Controlled Abciximab and Device Investigation to Lower Late Angioplasty Complications
CAPRIE	Clopidogrel versus Aspirin in Patients at Risk for Ischemic Events
CARE	Cholesterol and Recurrent Events
CCB	calcium channel blocker
CCP	Cooperative Cardiovascular Project
CHARISMA	Clopidogrel for High Atherothrombotic Risk and Ischemic Stabilization, Management, and Avoidance
CHD	coronary heart disease
CHF	congenital heart failure
CI	confidence interval
CREDO	Clopidogrel for Reduction of Events During Observation
CRP	C-reactive protein
CURE	Clopidogrel in Unstable Angina to Prevent Recurrent Events
CVA	cardiovascular accident
DAG	diacylglycerol
DAIS	Diabetes Atherosclerosis Intervention Study
DBP	diastolic blood pressure
DCCT	Diabetes Control and Complications Trial
DIGAMI	Diabetes Mellitus, Insulin Glucose Infusion in Acute Myocardial Infarction

EAST	Emory Angioplasty Surgery Trial
EC	endothelial cell
ECG	electrocardiogram
EF	ejection fraction
eNOS	endothelial nitric oxide synthase
EPCR	endothelial protein C receptor
EPIC	Evaluation of c7E3 for the Prevention of Ischemic Complications
EPILOG	Evaluation of PTCA to Improve Long-term Outcome with Abciximab GPIIb/IIIa Blockade
EPISTENT	Evaluation of Platelet IIb/IIIa Inhibitor for Stenting Trial
ERACI-II	Argentine Randomized Study of Coronary Angioplasty with Stenting versus Coronary Artery Bypass Surgery in Patients with Multiple-vessel Disease
ESRD	endstage renal disease
ESSENCE	Efficacy and Safety of Subcutaneous Enoxaparin in Non-Q-wave Coronary Events Study
ET	endothelin
ETDRS	Early Treatment Diabetic Retinopathy Study
FACET	Fosinopril versus Amlodipine Cardiovascular Events Randomized Trial
FBF	forearm blood flow
FMD	flow-mediated dilation
FPA	fibrinopeptide A
FPB	fibrinopeptide B
FPG	fasting plasma glucose
FREEDOM	Future Revascularization Evaluation in Patients with Diabetes Mellitus

FRISC	Fragmin and Fast Revascularization during Instability in Coronary Artery Disease
FTT	Fibrinolytic Therapy Trialists'
GFR	glomerular filtration rate
GISSI	Gruppo Italiano per lo Studio Della Sopravvivenza Nell'Infarto Miocardico
Gla	γ-carboxyglutamic acid
GP	glycoprotein
GUSTO	Global Utilization of Streptokinase and Tissue Plasminogen Activator for Occluded Coronary Arteries
Hb	hemoglobin
HDL	high-density lipoprotein
HERO	Hirulog and Early Reperfusion or Occlusion
HMG-CoA	3-hydroxy-3-methylglutaryl-coenzyme A
HOMO	Homeostasis Model Assessment
HOPE	Heart Outcomes Prevention Evaluation
HOT	Hypertension Optimal Treatment
IDNT	Irbesartan Diabetic Nephropathy Trial
IGT	impaired glucose tolerance
IL	interleukin
IMT	intimal medial thickness
INDIANA	Individual Data Analysis of Antihypertensive Drug Interventions
IRMA II	Irbesartan in Patients with Type II Diabetes and Microalbuminuria
ISR	in-stent restenosis
JNC	Joint National Commission
LDL	low-density lipoprotein
LIFE	Losartan Intervention for Endpoint Reduction in Hypertension

LIPS	Lescol Intervention Prevention Study
LMWH	low-molecular weight heparin
LPa	lipoprotein a
LV	left ventricular
LVEF	left ventricular ejection fraction
LVH	left ventricular hypertrophy
MACE	major adverse cardiac event
MARVAL	Microalbuminuria Reduction with Valsartan
MATH	Modern Approach to the Treatment of Hypertension
MI	myocardial infarction
MIAMI	Metoprolol in Acute Myocardial Infarction
MICRO-HOPE	Microalbuminuria, Cardiovascular and Renal Outcomes Substudy of the Heart Outcomes Prevention Efficacy
MIRACL	Myocardial Ischemia Reduction with Aggressive Lowering
MOCHA	Multicenter Oral Carvedilol Heart Failure Assessment
MRFIT	Multiple Risk Factor Intervention Trial
NCEP/ATP	National Cholesterol Education Program Adult Treatment Panel
NHLBI	National Heart, Lung, and Blood Institute
NHANES	National Health and Nutrition Examination Survey
NO	nitric oxide
NRMI	National Registry of Myocardial Infarction
NSTE-ACS	non-ST-segment elevation ACS
O^{2-}	superoxide anion
OASIS	Organization to Assess Strategies for Ischemic Syndromes

OGTT	oral glucose tolerance testing
OR	odds ratio
PAD	peripheral arterial disease
PAI	plasminogen activator inhibitor
PAMI	Primary Angioplasty in Myocardial Infarction
PAR	proteinase-activated receptor
PCI	percutaneous coronary intervention
PDT	platelet-dependent thrombosis
PGI_2	prostacyclin
PKC	protein kinase C
PPAR	Prevention of Adverse Events following Percutaneous Coronary Revascularization
PRISM-PLUS	Platelet Receptor Inhibition in Ischemic Syndrome Management in Patients Limited by Unstable Signs and Symptoms
PTCA	percutaneous transluminal coronary angioplasty
PVD	peripheral vascular disease
RAPPORT	ReoPro and Primary PTCA Organization and Randomized Trial
RAVEL	Randomized Study with the Sirolimus-eluting Velocity Balloon-expandable Stent
REIN	Ramipril Efficacy in Nephropathy
RENAAL	Reduction of Endpoints with the Angiotensin II Antagonist Losartan
RR	relative risk
SAVE	Survival and Ventricular Enlargement
SBP	systolic blood pressure
SHEP	Systolic Hypertension in the Elderly Program
sICAM	soluble intercellular adhesion molecule
SIRUS	North American Sirolimus-Eluting Stent

SK	streptokinase
SMBG	self-monitoring blood glucose
SNP	single nucleotide polymorphism
SOS	Stent or Surgery
STEMI	acute ST-elevation MI
sVCAM	soluble vascular cell adhesion molecule
Syst-Eur	Systolic Hypertension in Europe
T1DM	type 1 diabetes mellitus
T2DM	type 2 diabetes mellitus
TACTICS-TIMI	Treat Angina with Aggrastat and Determine the Cost of Therapy with an Invasive or Conservative Strategy
TAFI	thrombin-activatable fibrinolysis inhibitor
TAMI	Thrombolysis and Angioplasty in Myocardial Infarction
TARGET	do Tirofiban and ReoPro give similar Efficacy Trial
TF	tissue factor
TFPI	tissue factor pathway inhibitor
TG	triglyceride
TGF	transforming growth factor
TIMI	Thrombolysis in Myocardial Infarction
tPA	tissue-type plasminogen activator
TVR	target vessel revascularization
TZD	thiazolidinedione
UAE	urinary albumin excretion
UAER	urinary albumin excretion rate
UFH	unfractionated heparin
UKPDS	United Kingdom Prospective Diabetes Study
uPA	urokinase-type plasminogen activator

USRDS	United States Renal Data System
VA-HIT	Veterans Affairs Cooperative Studies Program High-density Lipoprotein Intervention Trial
VCAM	vascular cell adhesion molecule
VEGF	vascular endothelial growth factor
VLDL	very low-density lipoprotein
vWF	von Willebrand factor
WHO	World Health Organization

Index

A

α_2-antiplasmin 51–53
α-linoleic acid 91, 92
ABCD, trial 84, 122–123
abciximab 34, 136, 139, 141, 159, 167–169
ACE inhibitors
    captopril 9, 101, 122
    enalapril 84, 123
    fosinopril 77, 122
    lisinopril 77, 79, 85
    ramipril 9, 76–79, 101, 124, 148–149
ACS, adjunctive medical therapy for patients with diabetes and 141–150
    ACE inhibitors 147–148
    antithrombin therapy 143–146
        unfractionated heparin 143–144
        low molecular-weight heparin 144
        direct thrombin inhibitors 145–146
    beta-blockers 146–147
    intravenous GPIIb/IIIa receptor inhibitors for NSTE-ACS 141–142
    lipid-lowering therapy 148–150
    oral antiplatelet therapy 143
        aspirin 143
        clopidogrel 143